❧ *The New Cancer Survivors*

The New Cancer Survivors

Living with Grace, Fighting with Spirit

Natalie Davis Spingarn

The Johns Hopkins University Press
Baltimore and London

Note to the reader: This book is not intended to provide medical or legal advice for people with cancer. The services of a competent professional should be obtained whenever medical, legal, or other specific advice is needed.

The Johns Hopkins University Press
2715 North Charles Street
Baltimore, Maryland 21218-4363
www.press.jhu.edu

Library of Congress Cataloging-in-Publication Data will be found at the end of this book.
A catalog record for this book is available from the British Library.

ISBN 0-8018-6266-3
ISBN 0-8018-6267-1 (pbk.)

"I reason, Earth is short . . ." is reprinted by permission of the publishers and the Trustees of Amherst College from *The Poems of Emily Dickinson,* Thomas H. Johnson, ed., Cambridge, Mass.: The Belknap Press of Harvard University Press, copyright © 1951, 1955, 1979, 1983 by the President and Fellows of Harvard College.

Excerpt from "East Coker" in *Four Quartets,* copyright © 1943 by T. S. Eliot and renewed 1971 by Esme Valerie Eliot, reprinted by permission of Harcourt Brace & Company.

"Ode to my Cancer-Ridden Body" from *An Unfinished Life,* copyright © 1990 by Barbara Boggs Sigmund, reprinted by permission of the Arts Council of Princeton.

"Watching the Moon" from *The Ink Dark Moon* by Jane Hirshfield and Mariko Aratami, copyright © 1990 by Jane Hirshfield and Mariko Aratami, reprinted by permission of Vintage Books, a division of Random House Inc.

"Gravy" by Raymond Carver in *A New Path to the Waterfall,* copyright © 1989 by The Estate of Raymond Carver, reprinted by permission of Grove/Atlantic, Inc.

For my fellow survivors, past, present, and future:
Be strong, Be Strong, and let us Strengthen One Another.

—adapted from II Samuel 10:12 and I Chronicles 19:13

❧ Contents

✿ *Preface*

Living is what this book is about, not dying—except insofar as dying has, in the past few years, become a part of the natural process of living. Some of the "cancer books" now happily available on bookshop and library shelves tell personal tales of great fortitude; others describe special cures ranging from vitamin therapy and mind control to shark cartilage. Still others provide a wealth of material on different aspects of survivorship, like the prevention of cancer and its recurrence.

This book takes the matter beyond the how-to and personal story approaches to address realistically the paramount issues for those of us who are, after all, still alive: living with a serious, scary illness, and dealing with what that illness brings in both our medical and nonmedical lives, without becoming a burden to ourselves and those around us. It is neither a case history nor a medical tome. Rather, it is the distillation of the experiences of the author, who is also a health care writer, and of others who have been through it all.

It aims to be useful to all survivors and to those who are help- ing them. And though it does not try to "put a happy face" onto painful human and social problems, it seeks to serve as a matter- of-fact, upbeat gift for the new or seasoned survivor.

For much of my adult life, I have written about health care and social policy for newspapers and magazines. After I fell ill with cancer in the early 1970s, I began to write in terms of my own experience, particularly in the *Washington Post*'s "Outlook" section. In other ways, I opened up to tell my story, in, for example, a script titled "A Different Kind of Life," which aired on the Jim Lehrer public television series *U.S. Chronicle* (1981), in which I appeared as one of three women with cancer.

I was struck by the response. You can write the most well reasoned, thoroughly documented third-person story in the world, and people may or may not notice it. But write personally about yourself, and the phone will ring off the hook for days, sometimes for months. Though people hunger for authoritative health information, they respond most strongly to stories about individual human beings.

So I decided to expand what I had begun and address the relatively new problems of the patient who is, thanks to modern medical science and new feelings of empowerment, hanging in there with an illness—particularly cancer—that once evoked only submission or surrender. In my book *Hanging in There: Living Well on Borrowed Time,* which first appeared in 1982, I wove my own cancer experiences and those of others in my shoes in with the psychosocial and medical issues confronting survivors.

The welcome extended to this book surpassed my most optimistic expectations. Survivors particularly have told me that it has helped them in innumerable ways to chart their journeys, whether that meant communicating with their doctors in a more assertive, constructive way, or solving an insurance problem, or adjusting their emotional approach to a recurrence (don't forget that the word *survivor* throughout this book means someone who has simply heard a doctor say "You have cancer," someone living with a diagnosis of cancer, no matter if that be for five minutes or five or fifty years). These survivors, their friends and families, and, importantly, their professional caretakers have given the book a long shelf life. The National Coalition for Cancer Survivorship (NCCS) has labeled it a "classic" in its field, while a former editor of the *New York Times Book Review,* Anatole Broyard, called it one of the better nonfiction books about being sick.

In the past few years, with medicine and the world about it undergoing seismic changes, survivors have repeatedly asked me to update *Hanging in There;* most recently, one such person— a feisty paralegal—phoned to say how she had found my book in her public library: "This phone call is a *hug*," she told me. Gradually, as hospital and office treatments changed, and as survivors gained a more powerful voice, I listened to them more carefully. Who would have thought, for instance, in 1982 when I wrote about my own hospitalization, that in less than two decades the week-long hospital stay would have vanished and that survivors would be experiencing "drive through" cancer surgeries, returning to their homes after mastectomies in a day or less, unsure as to how to deal with a tangle of tubes draining their wounds?

Clearly, we survivors live in a different world. In 1982, the number of living Americans with a history of cancer was some 3 million; now it is estimated at more than 8 million. Then, survivors had not organized, and the word *survivorship* had not been coined; now support and advocacy groups abound on both local and national levels. Then, I was a reluctant participant in occasional hospital support groups; now I have invested years of time and effort in the survivorship cause—as a leader of both a nationwide advocacy group and an international patient's network. On a warm fall day in 1998 it felt good to be marching with an estimated two hundred thousand other survivors and their supporters on the Washington Mall, demanding "No More Cancer!"

Though cancer has not been "cured," its treatment has become much more effective, and attitudes toward those of us who live with serious disease have become more enlightened. Nevertheless, we still live with a variety of problems, and new changes in the health care delivery system have produced complicated and confusing choices. When the Johns Hopkins University Press proposed a new edition of *Hanging in There*, I was ready—even eager—to sign on to do it. In the writing, it has turned into a new book with a title more appropriate to the times: *The New Cancer Survivors: Living with Grace, Fighting with Spirit*. Though this much larger book contains a great deal of research, I did not want to weigh the reader down with tedious footnotes. Instead, I have chosen to end the book with notes keyed to individual pages to guide readers through the material and direct those who wish to additional information and resources.

I cannot begin to thank adequately the cooperative people at the Press, especially the talented Jacqueline Wehmueller, who has served as an ideal editor, supportive yet diligent and constructively critical. In a time when her equals are fast disappearing, she doesn't miss a trick. The Commonwealth Fund and Robert Wood Johnson Foundation provided the necessary support for me to undertake a challenging job; I am especially grateful to the Fund's Karen Davis and RWJ's Frank Karel, who believed that I could do it; to the NCCS staff, who facilitated the process; and to the longtime director of the National Health Policy Forum, Judith Miller Jones, who encouraged me to seek research and writing support grants.

I benefited from the help of a fine group of Georgetown University and other students who served as my research assistants, keeping me afloat in a sea of on- and off-line information provided by experts and survivors who wanted to help. Special thanks are due Ann Broeker, Deborah Landes, Nathan Townsend, and Eric Anderson (who deserves extra kudos for his diligent work), as well as Jenny Hopkins, Susan Rohol, and Courtney O'Donnell. For her experienced eye in preparing the manuscript for publication and composing the index, my heartfelt thanks to Laurie MacDonald Brumberg. The host of experts, some of whose names appear in this book, range from social scientists like Judith Feder, psychologist Julia Rowland, and anthropologist Betty Randall to physicians Phil Cohen and Kathy Alley and health care attorney Diann Austin; all were generous with their time and comments. Fellow survivor Eleanor Nealon helped guide me along the sometimes obscure pathways at the National Cancer Institute.

And of course my family, especially my husband, Jerry, deserves credit for putting up with me as I strove to weave fifteen years of progress in cancer survivorship into and beyond the older text. Though I made every effort to keep up to date as I finished writing in late 1998, both science and survivorship may occasionally have outpaced me. I cherish a hope that in the next fifteen years, and surely in the next century, the unhappy disease at the root of such projects will be gone and that another edition—by myself or some other author/survivor—will not be necessary.

❧ *The New Cancer Survivors*

1 ∞ *Hanging In There*

"How are you?" people ask me, still rather shakily, knowing that I have been treated for repeated bouts with metastatic breast cancer (and a few other diseases as well) since 1974. "Hanging in there," I reply.

The statistics show that more and more of us are doing just that. In the early 1900s, few cancer patients had any hope of survival. In the 1930s, according to the American Cancer Society (ACS), fewer than one in five was alive five years after treatment; in the 1960s it was one in three. Today—in 1998—about 491,400 Americans, or four out of ten people who get this disease, will survive five years or more—a gain that represents more than 91,000 men, women, and children each year.

When you adjust this "observed" survival rate for the normal hazards of aging (like dying of heart disease or accidents), far more than half of us will survive. And that "relative" rate, now 58 percent, is edging upward and should continue to do so according to the upbeat "report card" released in March 1998 by the ACS, National Cancer Institute (NCI), and Centers for Disease Control and Prevention (CDC). This report showed that between 1990 and 1995 both the number of new cancer cases and the number of deaths from the disease had begun to drop, in a sharp reversal of the steady increase observed through most of the century.

"I think it's going our way," NCI director Dr. Richard Klausner told me in an interview several months after the report. "It remains incremental, but the numbers that give us some measure of the cancer burden—incidence rates, mortality rates, survival rates, attempts to quantify quality of life—are beginning to move in the right direction."

According to Dr. Klausner, a formidable but refreshing young scientist/administrator who likes to be called "Rick" and seldom wears a jacket and tie to the office, we (meaning researchers) "have to be humble" about how much credit to take for these numbers showing a dramatic reversal of a twenty-year trend, a reversal that he attributes in great measure to better prevention and treatment. Still, he feels the statistical gains will accelerate as the effects of screening (in breast cancer, for instance) begin to kick in and we reach "a much better place than we have ever been in terms of our understanding of cancer and the proximity of that understanding to intervention."

As we near the century's end, cancer survivors have reason to join in the rising tide of optimism. Almost every day, it seems, the news brings fresh reports of potential treatments and new ways of dealing with cancer—the identification of still another cancer gene, which might someday be translated into gene therapy; trials of known agents like tamoxifen in the possible prevention of disease; and completely new approaches aiming not to bombard existing tumors with chemotherapy but to cut off their nourishing blood supply (angiogenesis), causing them to starve and die. Asked on the public radio program "All Things Considered" how I felt about this "discovery," already succeeding with mice, I replied, "Bittersweet"—tremendously excited for the people who would probably benefit from it but sad that such progress did not come in time to save me pain and precious body parts and, for countless friends, to save life itself.

Of course research in the laboratory, until it can be applied, saves mice, not men. Still, we are seeing a significant increase in new ideas entering clinical trials; the number of new drugs or other agents being tested has risen five- to sixfold in just ten years. And we are beginning to see one transformation we've really been waiting for: the moving of treatment and prevention approaches "from empirical to rational." This means that instead of trying toxic drugs as the doctors did with me—first in this combination, then in that, hit or miss—they will be able to treat different cancers in a more specific way, according to rational designs.

Until this day comes, I will cling to my healthy disrespect for statistics. I know from my own experience working in government, as a journalist and as a sometimes public relations flack, that statistics can be used selectively to prove a point. I wonder, since I am alive almost a quarter century after my first mastectomy, and since I have changed treatment sites several times, how many times I have shown up in some biostatistician's "cured" columns, though I have had recurrences and honestly do not belong there.

I know, too, how complicated, confusing, and controversial has been the success of our country's long war on cancer—a war currently funded at more than two billion dollars a year. I know how stubbornly some cancers—notably cancer of the lung and pancreas (to which I lost my beloved older sister)—have refused to yield to scientific progress. I know that well over half a million people—some fifteen hundred women, men, and children a day—will die of cancer this year. Still, as Dr. Klausner points out, remarkable progress has been made through medical sciences' "empirical" approaches, especially in the improvement of childhood and testicular cancers; more personally, 82 percent of us breast cancer patients are surviving five years or more, and my son, a mathematics professor, is thriving almost a decade after a difficult bout with Hodgkin's disease (for which the survival rate is now more than 95 percent).

And as our nation gets tougher in its approach to tobacco products, even recalcitrant lung cancer mortality rates have begun to creep downward. So have rates for cancer of the oral cavity, the other major cancer I have suffered (without, I must add, exposure to the main risk factors—it is more than thirty years since I've smoked, and I've never been a heavy drinker). I say "major" cancer because the official numbers do not even include the many basal and squamous cancers my dermatologist constantly freezes or cuts off my skin (for this, I do plead guilty; only in recent years have I stopped the sunbathing I love and been meticulous about covering myself with sunscreen).

Keep in mind: Neither we survivors nor our official statistical observers are as hung up on the word *cure* as we used to be. The ACS says we can be considered "cured" when we have no signs of disease and our life expectancy is the same as that of a person who never had cancer. Though the five-year rate is used for purposes of comparison, we all know it varies dramatically among cancers and even among people who have those cancers. No person is a statistic; he or she is a human being, each different from the other, who may or may not fall into the median on any statistical curve.

Recognizing the growing survivor population and its unfortunate high risk not only for serious hanging-in problems but for second and even third cancers, the NCI has launched several significant survivorship initiatives: the Office of Liaison Activities, a central, two-way point of contact for cancer advocacy organizations that has created mechanisms whereby survivors can have a voice in shaping NCI decision making, and the Office of Cancer Survivorship, which looks at therapies in terms of their impact on both survival and quality of survival. As Dr. Klausner put it, "We need to design and redesign clinical trials to ask questions about not just 'Do you survive?' but 'How?'"

What good news! Ten years ago, when I went out to Bethesda to interview the NCI official responsible for survivorship matters for the first issue of the National Coalition for Cancer Survivorship (NCCS) *Networker*, I found the very word *survivorship* unfamiliar and less than 1 percent of the total NCI budget being spent on what was then called "rehabilitation and continuing care" research. And when I appeared on a Pennsylvania talk show, a lady in the audience raised her hand. Why, she asked, since I walked, talked, and had flown to Pittsburgh to appear on television, was I not "well?" I explained that people used to feel a person who developed cancer would either die or be cured. But I was neither, really, since I was still with her on this earth and no doctor had ever labeled me "cured." I told her I preferred to say I was "hanging in there"— part of the survivorship picture then unfamiliar to the public.

Appearing recently on the nationwide Larry King show, my friend Ellen Stovall, the NCCS executive director, pointed out that the notion of "cure" implies a measure of permanence that may or may not be realistic. Said Ellen, a twenty-seven-year, two-time Hodgkin's disease survivor who is as compelling as she is endearing: "Hams are for curing. People are for surviving."

Be that as it may, I believe what I see and hear, and I know that it's not just that survivors are hanging in for longer periods of time as we approach the new century. It is that they are doing so with style. Most of them are living what our doctors call "quality lives." As my lifelong friend Betty Slater, a California writer who had the lumpectomy with radiation to achieve a breast cancer "cure" more than a decade ago, puts it: "I'm not surprised when people live on like us, leading good gutsy lives; I'm surprised when they do not."

True; the new breed of survivors is, by and large, an extraordinary lot. I met such women and men en masse for the first time when I went to Albuquerque, New Mexico, in the late 1980s, to keynote the NCCS's first national assembly. I had expected another meeting, another speech, a stalwart but perhaps sad audience full of questions about how I felt when I was first diagnosed with cancer, or what treatments I had taken, and which physicians and hospitals I had consulted.

Instead I found a gathering of people who had been through the trials of the cancer experience and had come out punching. I found *them* the teachers and myself the learner. Hopping on one of those little Toonerville trolleys to Olde Towne, I sat next to another conference participant, a slight lady of my general vintage with a deceptively soft, sweet southern drawl who introduced herself as Sally Henderson, executive director of CAnCare in Charlotte, North Carolina.

We fell to chatting, and I asked, "What's with your health?" It took us all the way downtown and back for her to tell me about her four cancers and the feisty, intelligent way she had dealt with them. She had bilateral breast cancer in 1973, then colon cancer in 1979, followed by melanoma of the eye and lung cancer. "Not much left," joked this short, energetic widow, who confessed to walking three and a half miles a day in addition to working and, importantly, falling in love.

Sally enjoyed discussing cancer problems with other survivors like John, a golf-playing accountant whose leg had been amputated at the hip six years before. As she put it, "We're able to talk about it now; we slug it out in the open." And she continued to do that until she left us, after nearly a quarter century of survivorship.

Other survivors I met during that landmark week in Albuquerque remain my mentors. For example, I've watched Susan Leigh, a nurse who had seen tough service in Vietnam (and whose Hodgkin's disease is suspected to have been caused by Agent Orange), make what she calls a "180-degree turn"—from a depressed patient isolated in the Arizona desert, and afraid even to discuss her disease, to an outspoken consultant. Despite two new (breast and bladder) cancers, she travels the country beating the survivorship drums as she talks primarily to nursing audiences about issues like fear of recurrence, the late effects of harsh treatments, and the change in doctor/patient relationships in the past decade or so, "from paternalism to partnership."

I see and meet and read about survivors like Sally and Susie every day. Indeed, they seem a new breed. They expect to survive. Instead of resigning themselves to their fates, many of them, after an initial rough shocked period, set about fighting for their lives, searching for new treatments, investigating new ways, working hard for the right to enjoy "quality time." Seldom do they hide any more, even if they have suffered disfigurement or disabilities.

Now more men swell their numbers, talking about their illnesses, exchanging information about treatment options and experimental possibilities. Whether it be Buster Jackson, the smiling general factotum at Scheele's, our corner grocery store, combing the neighborhood for advice on how to deal with his two-year-old prostate cancer (and finding it from an eminent research physician), or swashbuckling retired General "Stormin' Norman" Schwarzkopf spreading the word for men to have their prostates checked, they are out of the closet. And they feel better for it.

"My doctor says I won't die until I finish paying his bill," Buster told me a few months ago as I picked up my frozen peas and croissants at Scheele's, "and that should be a long, long time."

Buster feels lucky. Not only is he blessed with a loving, supportive family and a sunny disposition, but he is well insured under his wife's federal health plan. Others are not so lucky: patients whose particularly lethal cancers gave them little time or little chance to fight; people whose lack of resources or education prevents them from taking advantage of new approaches. Still others—and they seem a diminishing bunch—try to forget the whole thing or prefer, for whatever reasons, to take the stance of a dependent invalid.

Of course, all of us go through tough times at the beginning of our illnesses—and each time we are diagnosed anew. I remember a story one of my doctors told me in the late 1970s about a woman whose breast cancer had spread—or metastasized—to a spot in her back, much like mine. She was roughing it in Iceland and feeling better. A certain upbeat swing to that tale appealed to me; it made me feel I, too, could regain a measure of control; something could be done to help me, even if it meant formidable treatment.

It takes time to gain confidence and to learn certain ways, techniques if you will, that help us grow stronger—to become not victims, or even "patient" patients, but impatient survivors. When I first saw large numbers of little bald-headed, scrawny children with cancer at Memorial Sloan-Kettering Cancer Center, I thought their hanging-in problems were pitiful but different from mine. Because they had lived shorter lives, they had a different perspective. Their lot seemed unfair, too, but I felt that since they had made less investment in the future, they generally had fewer potential dividends to lose—like my yearning to have grandchildren and then see them grow up.

Perhaps, I thought, I had more in common with the parents of those poignant little people, who could seem so unlovable just when they needed love most. After all, these moms and dads, like me, were in danger of losing one of their most important life investments, some of their own most cherished future dividends. But gradually I came to feel that though the hanging-in children's problems differed from my own, they resembled them as well.

In a picture book, *There Is a Rainbow behind Every Dark Cloud,* a group of California children with cancer wrote about the choices they had made to help themselves feel happy "inside," despite what's going on "outside." They said you can speak up and say what's on your mind; you can cry; you can be mad at the world; and you can be afraid of death. You can use your imagination to fight disease; for them, this meant accepting their situation and expressing their feelings about it in drawings and through dreams, as well as conversation. I, too, chose to make myself feel better "inside" by trying matter-of-factly to accept what had happened and by speaking and writing forthrightly about my disease.

It may have taken me longer than the "Rainbow Kids," but like them, I learned important survival skills as I went along, certain ways of eliciting different behavior from friends and relatives. For the kids, this meant depending on other children who, as they put it, talk the same language and so could be more helpful to them than adults. For me, particularly when I have been in active treatment, this meant that though I am basically an independent person, I had to accept a measure of dependence on others; I needed friends to drive me around or bring me supper. Later it meant talking to my fellow survivors, sharing joys and sorrows, and, still later, learning assertiveness and working together on survivorship issues.

The other side of the coin did not escape the California children. They pointed out that when other kids tease you, you can either pay no attention, fight them, or choose to see that they are really scared. I, too, found that when my adult friends avoided or acted strangely toward "cancerous" me, I could ignore them, or confront them with their deeds and words, or speak to them in an understanding way, choosing to see that they were really scared. At one party, after harsh chemotherapy treatments began to make my hair fall out, I found myself talking to two women. One complimented me on my hairdo. "Oh, thank you," I replied. "It's a wig." The women disappeared into the canapes.

I had confronted them, in a way. But I chose to understand their fears.

Importantly, the kids who saw a rainbow behind every cloud acknowledged the necessity, as one social worker I consulted put it, to "place yourself existentially"—try to figure out the meaning of living. They spoke of the power of love and of prayer, of letting go of the past, forgiving everyone, not being afraid of the future, and knowing that this instant is the time that counts.

I, too, have found that cancer forced me to view my life more critically and intensively, through the eye of a needle as it were, to sort out what I want to do from what I do not and then, insofar as I can, to go ahead and do it. These children helped themselves by placing everything in God's hands; though I have become more comfortable with this approach as I've lived longer, I have helped myself lose my fear primarily by working—particularly with other survivors—by keeping alive my hope in the future, and by continuing to learn and develop a talent for life and to search for its deeper meaning.

With the passage of time, with the conquest of setbacks, we survivors are able to move ahead and gain strength. With the increase in our ability to take a nap, or work shorter hours, or complain to the doctor when necessary, we gain confidence. As one hospital social worker who has worked with cancer patients once put it, her "older" survivors (in years since diagnosis) used to consider their return to a functional life "magic." Now, the "younger" ones simply ask, "When do we begin fitting in again?"

Our doctors say they want to help us lead "normal" lives. "Normal Shmormal," wrote journalist Stewart Alsop in *Stay of Execution*, now dated but still one of the very good books about a struggle with cancer. More recently Wendy Harpham, the talented physician-writer who has suffered three setbacks in her battle with non-Hodgkin's lymphoma, coined the term "new normal" as the state in which cancer becomes a manageable part of daily life. In *When a Parent Has Cancer*, this Texas dynamo teaches parents that the greatest gift we can give our children—of any age—is not protection but the confidence and tools to cope and grow with what life has to offer them.

Part of the "new normal" we survivors live with is the persistent knowledge of our own mortality. "Background Music," Alsop called that knowledge, and with it comes a loss of that wonderful ignorance in which we never worried about putting off a trip to Greece, or remodeling the basement, or trying a new line of work or play, be it white-water rafting out west, or playing tennis, or trying one's hand, finally, at fiction.

I have found no skill more important (no matter how it is gained) than the ability to believe in my survival. For this I have been dependent on my fellow human beings—whether family and friends or doctors and nurses. I have been dependent on how they talk and deal with me and on what they give me, be it comfort or new medical knowledge, as much as on some higher force. I have needed them to reinforce the hope that sustains me; I only hope to have more time to continue giving something back to all of them and to future cancer survivors.

My spirits were lifted by a talk with Andrea DiLorenzo, a fourteen-year survivor who has suffered two bouts with breast and one with ovarian cancer and is now adopting two "older" children. "Time was slipping by," she told me. "We wanted the kids now. After all I'm here and I'm alive. The decision feels good; it feels wonderful to me and my husband too." (About Andrea, more later.)

In the same way, Bethine Church once observed that I was quite right in feeling that "the cancer twilight zone . . . is a world that other people haven't lived in." Describing the late Senator Frank Church's fight with cancer thirty years before and their feeling then that he had only six months to live, she said that forever after, her husband had been a different person. It had been somehow easier for him to do the things that needed to be done and let the things that did not matter go. We are all different people during, and after, an experience with cancer.

This background music—even in our "new normal" hanging-in years—forces most of us toward a search for meaning. Some find strength in a deepened religious belief—in a new relationship with their God or, like me, in an intensification of a faltering old one. As the line between science and religion has grown increasingly fuzzy, it seems to me that those men and women who have found a strong, clear spiritual faith of any kind are lucky indeed— whether it be in or outside a traditional religion.

After all my survivor years, I still spend a good deal of time weaving my thoughts together, trying to figure out the meaning of the time we have been given on this earth. But no one, certainly not I, could have put the difficulties of doing so as succinctly as the solitary poet Emily Dickinson:

> I reason, Earth is short—
> And Anguish—absolute—
> And many hurt,
> But, what of that?
>
> I reason, we could die—
> The best Vitality
> Cannot excel Decay,
> But, what of that?
>
> I reason, that in Heaven—
> Somehow, it will be even—
> Some new Equation, given—
> But, what of that?

2 ❧ The Bad News

The wounded surgeon plies the steel
That questions the distempered part;
Beneath the bleeding hands we feel
The sharp compassion of the healer's art
Resolving the enigma of the fever chart.
                    —T. S. Eliot, "East Coker"

The phone rings. "Is this Toots?" asks a distraught voice. I think
it must be someone who knew me, but not very well, long ago.
She pronounced my childhood nickname with a short *o* (as in
"Tootsie Roll"), while my family and close old friends use a long
o (as in "loose").

Right. A friend of an old friend was calling me as a supposed
fountain of knowledge about breast cancer. She had had previous
biopsies that had proved benign. Tomorrow she was scheduled
for another biopsy, of a particularly thick, threatening lump. She
understood I had been through similar experiences. What did I
think; what kind of operation should she have if she got bad
news? Had she chosen her doctor correctly?

I helped her as much as I could. I did not know her physician
and advised a consultation at a comprehensive cancer center if
the lump proved malignant and she was still unsure as to how to
proceed. I warned her not to delay: even though some tumors
grow very slowly, some sprout before your eyes. (*To conduct an
effective transaction with the environment,* says the coping literature, *the patient must secure adequate information.*) And I

thought how much had happened in the world of breast cancer—
how much progress had been made—since my first mastectomy.

Late summer 1974. I had been in Bucharest reporting the World
Population Conference; a week later in Jerusalem, my husband
and I were exploring Israel. I remember how big and hard the
lump felt when I found it rubbing the washcloth over my right
breast in the shower, but Jerry was reassuring, as usual. Admit-
tedly, it was there, he said as he touched it tenderly, if a bit gin-
gerly, but I had had lumps for ten years on and off and had taken
them to the doctor; they had proved benign. Why should this one
be different?

So I took a tour of Hadassah Hospital, as scheduled, and back
in the hotel suggested to Jerry, "They're so smart here, perhaps I
should show them the lump?" But he pointed out I did not want
to be hospitalized in a foreign country, away from friends and
family, and we went on to Spain as planned, where we visited
our old friends Len and Betty Slater in Menorca. As we strolled
through that quaint island countryside, checkerboarded with
stone walls and white cottages, I started to tell Betty about the
damned lump I kept feeling in my breast. But I stopped because I
thought it might prove to be just another cyst, and I did not want
to worry anyone needlessly.

Home again, I called my cancer specialist, Dr. Calvin Klopp,
and visited his office that same September week. As my husband
had reminded me abroad, I had gone to this calm, efficient surgeon for more than a decade because I suffered from what was
then called chronic fibrocystic disease (lumpy breasts); I felt
comfortable with him and trusted him. He had sent me to the
hospital several times for biopsies and had aspirated numerous
cysts in his office. If a lump came back after aspiration, he took
it out even if it proved benign (too much activity there); if it was
hard, questionable, he removed it as a matter of course.

Somehow, both Dr. Klopp and I seemed to sense a difference
this time; the lump had grown fast since he had examined me
only a few months before. He said I'd go into the hospital the
next week for my biopsy, and he gave me a choice, the first of
many survivorship choices that lay ahead. I could give him per-

mission to proceed as he saw fit; do the biopsy, and if the results
were benign, fine, he would sew me up again; if not, he would go
ahead and perform the sort of mastectomy he felt best for me
(then called the "one-stage procedure"). My other choice would
be to have the biopsy and let him close the wound and we could
discuss the results. If he found a malignancy, we would have a
week or two to decide together what sort of treatment or operation I would have (then the "two-stage operation").

That fall, two weeks before Betty Ford publicly acknowledged
her mastectomy, causing us to be engulfed in a tidal wave of
information, before Happy Rockefeller's operations and long
before mass breast cancer consciousness-raising, most of us
knew of no alternative to just placing yourself in your surgeon's
hands and telling him to do what's best for you—or at least what
he (then almost always a "he") would advise for his wife.

For a week, I did worry about the choice. I consulted my
internist, who advised me against the two-stage procedure; he
thought that the offer was a result of the increasing wave of mal-
practice suits against the profession. I talked to my sister, who
had had the operation; she credited women's-rights pressures
for the new patient participation. I called my physician-brother
in Baltimore; he said you would have to go to medical school,
perhaps complete residency training as a pathologist, to determine intelligently what treatment would be best for your own
particular cancer. You would have to know the meaning of the
type of cancer you suffered and its position in the breast.

I did not rush to the library to do research on mastectomies,
like a few rare women even then, including breast cancer advocate Rose Kushner (who, a bit earlier, had gone to great trouble
to get the two-stage operation in Buffalo, New York). But, wearing my reporter's hat, I talked to well-informed people and read
what I could get my hands on. For instance, I studied Dr. George
Crile's *What Women Should Know about the Breast Cancer
Controversy*, which dared suggest that mastectomy might not
be necessary in early breast cancer. And I watched his wife, the
writer Helga Sandburg, who had followed his advice, bare her
lumpectomy scar for a nationwide television audience to show
women they might fight cancer without losing a whole breast.

I felt calmer as I explored the alternatives. (Point number two from the coping literature: *Maintain emotional distress within tolerable limits and thereby maintain satisfactory physiological condition so as to process the information and act on it.*) At the end of what seemed a very long week, I chose the one-stage operation. It seemed my confidence in my doctor (who, I figured, did between two and three such operations a week—a total of almost five thousand over a thirty-year career) outweighed my faith in my own ability to choose losing my breast.

Dr. Klopp removed my breast and dissected almost all the axillary lymph nodes under my arm but preserved the chest muscles—a "modified radical" mastectomy, which an official National Institutes of Health (NIH) panel would soon (in 1979) recommend as a replacement for the disfiguring "Halstead radical"—a procedure that removed the underlying chest wall and was standard practice for some eighty years.

By the time a new "primary" cancer developed in my remaining breast six and a half years later, I—and breast cancer treatment—had begun to change. The one-stage operation was not offered and not even considered; indeed, as soon as I learned the bad news, I thought that I would probably ask for a breast-preserving lumpectomy with radiation. Why not? By then, evidence had begun to accumulate that the survival rates of patients with early breast cancer who had this procedure and of a similar group who had mastectomies were no different (a finding made official by another NIH panel in 1985).

Other procedures differed, too. Tissue could be removed by a needle from solid lumps, like fluid from a liquid-filled lump (not enough, however, could be extracted in my case to make a pathological decision, so a biopsy was necessary). There was more reliance on mammograms (X rays of the breast) and sonograms (pictures taken by sound waves). I was not put to sleep for my biopsy; it was done under local anesthetic in the hospital outpatient "In-and-Out" unit. The staff acted as though they were removing an ingrown toenail.

The diagnosis was not completed until the pathological slides had been sent out for expert consultation, a matter of a few weeks. During all this time I grew anxious and even angry at hospital bureaucrats for not responding promptly to the outside experts' demands for more slides. But I felt in control. We were proceeding step by step; *something* could be done. I grew more apprehensive with each passing day, but I did not panic. (Point number three: *Maintain autonomy and freedom of movement— taking care to avoid the feeling that there is either one right way or no way out.*)

Why, then, did I lose my remaining breast? Why did I not have the lumpectomy with radiation or, at the least, follow my second modified mastectomy with reconstruction so I would not need to wear falsies in my bra forever after?

Because between the two mastectomies, I had entered a different hanging-in world—the world of the metastatic cancer survivor. For two and a half years after the first operation, with its negative nodes and pronouncements of having "gotten it all," I had thought I was home free. I went about my business, a bit more bothered perhaps than the "normal" person about every little headache or belly cramp.

Spring 1977. My upper back started to ache. I felt as though I had played tennis too hard and strained my back muscles. I waited for the stabbing pain to go away, but it did not. I had a checkup; my internist said I probably was suffering the same arthritis that occasionally plagued my hip and knee, but, just the same, we'd do an X ray when I returned from a press club trip abroad. Between sightseeing forays in Portugal, I spent a good deal of time chasing electric transformers that would enable my trusty heating pad to work on European current and so comfort my aching back. Back home in Washington, I faced the X ray of my chest and spine, and another choice.

"You're not going to like this," my internist warned as he described the radiologist's finding. In brief, something had attacked my upper spine, and I had suffered a collapsed vertebra. Several more consultations and scans confirmed that my cancer had evidently metastasized (traveled to another part of my body), specifically to a small spot in my thoracic spine (T-6).

What to do? The sign on my surgeon's door announced his retirement in a few months. I had to find a new doctor. Should I head straight for a radiologist, or should I see an oncologist (a newer kind of cancer specialist who could give me chemotherapy if that proved necessary)? Should I try for admission to the National Cancer Institute (NCI), the government research center in nearby Bethesda, which at that time was looking for breast cancer patients like me, with one metastasis?

After my first mastectomy, I had undergone a series of body scans at the NCI and been pronounced fit. But now my surgeon advised against going to the NCI for care. Referring to the Pennsylvania-based physician who was honchoing the NCI's breast-research program, he warned, "You'll be taken care of by a computer in Pittsburgh." That was not quite accurate, but I understood what he meant. He wanted me to have more personal, flexible care than I would have had as a research subject, whereby my treatment would have been governed by a preset "protocol."

Some sort of wise genie stood up and whispered in my ear. I decided to go to a comprehensive cancer center for a consultation. There were none of these centers nearby at the time; now there are more than thirty scattered about the country (including two in the Washington/Baltimore area),* and they are focal points not only for research but for the broadest and most skilled care and training available. Any survivor—or any survivor who is adequately insured (see chapter 11)—can access them, at least for a consultation, and they will usually work with local community hospital staff to follow up.

But in the 1970s, I had to look to the New York area, where I still had family and friends. I called Dr. Lewis Thomas, the poet-physician who then headed the Memorial Sloan-Kettering Cancer Center in New York City, whom I had interviewed for a previous book. He did not horse around. "Come on up," he told me. "I'd like you to see Dr. Thomas Fahey. He's an internist, and a good one. We'll start there."

*For a list, and for other cancer-specific information, call the national Cancer Information Service at 1-800-4-CANCER, or call, using the telephone on a fax machine, the CancerFax automated information service at (301) 402-5874; Web users can access the same information at www. cancernet.nci.nih.gov.

I liked Tom Fahey right away. Not only was he a competent, humane internist, but he was also a skilled oncologist and endocrinologist. I could see on my first visit that he knew as much as there was to know about breast cancer at that point in time. And he was not above drawing the blood sample from my arm himself.

After going over me and my records thoroughly, he prescribed radiation to my back: "Let's sterilize that area first." After that, he strongly recommended an oophorectomy, which meant he wanted to take out my ovaries and give me an instant menopause (a bit past fifty, I still menstruated and showed little sign of stopping). I agreed to both.

I was to have six or seven weeks of radiation in Washington, D.C., with Tom Fahey continuing to supervise my treatment. Satisfied, I returned home. Again I felt better knowing something could be done—even if it turned out to be formidable treatment.

Each day, with weekends off, I lay alone in an isolated treatment room at George Washington University Hospital as a giant computerized machine targeted great bolts of radiation to the nasty spot on my spine, with technicians on the other side of the thick closed door talking to me occasionally by remote. A strange, scary experience, but it felt curative, if tiring. About two-thirds of the way through, I suffered one episode of traumatic discomfort, wherein I felt I was tumbling, like Humpty Dumpty, off the wall into some sort of dark abyss. That, too, passed, along with the fatigue.

Then I returned to Sloan-Kettering to begin the hormone treatment the doctors still think has kept me going over the long haul—first the oophorectomy, which gave me the chance, for the last time, to be taken care of by my mom in her comfortable home nearby. Whether it was her TLC or Dr. David Kinne's surgical skill, I recovered apace, and the hot menopausal flashes— which came quickly and violently—felt curative, too. If I needed hormonal treatment to help get rid of the cancer as the doctors seemed to feel, I was getting it, in spades.

Around that time, on a routine visit, Tom Fahey said in an off-hand way, "Something's come up in England; we want you to try it." So I became one of the first American patients to swallow antiestrogen tamoxifen pills. Again, I thought I was home free.

But in the spring of 1979 my left hip started to bother me. I bore with the pain for some weeks, trying once more to blame my arthritis. But the pain persisted and worsened. On a trip to Atlanta to see my mathematician son Jonathan, who had begun to teach at Georgia Tech, I had trouble moving my leg in and out of cars. I flew to New York, where Tom Fahey ordered a bone scan.

Later that evening, the oncologist told me both he and the radiologist were worried. My tumor had evidently spread; the bone scan showed a "hot" spot on my hip. Since tamoxifen had failed to control the cancer, he took me off it (later another anti-estrogen pill, a male hormone with the brand name Halotestin, was substituted). And he said he wanted first to radiate my hip and then to start me on chemotherapy: "If we continue to chase this thing only with radiation, we won't be doing anyone a favor."

I stayed first in the hospital and next in the then modest "hospital housing" for the hip radiation, which turned out to be no big deal (unlike the spot on my spine, this "hot" area was safely distant from sensitive nerves). I had begun to use a cane, but I was able to keep a May date to fly to Chicago and receive the American Psychiatric Association's annual Robert T. Morse Writers Award "for outstanding contributions to the public understanding of psychiatry."

It was a heady and somewhat unreal experience to leave the hospital and march in a wobbly way to a hotel platform to receive a bronze medal. (I had to return it temporarily so that the shrinks could correct their misspelling of the word *psychiatry!*) But I enjoyed myself. I got through the dinners and other convention trappings and made it back to Washington, via New York, to begin chemotherapy.

Late summer 1997. I am sitting in the comfortable office of Dr. Katherine Alley in Washington, D.C., discussing breast cancer treatment. "It's no wonder they did not recommend the lumpectomy or even mastectomy and reconstruction after your second breast surgery fifteen years ago," this snappy-looking surgeon told me, "with everything you had been through."

"You're right," I remembered. "Dr. Fahey knew the lumpectomy would have to be followed by radiation, and he said, 'We can't waste radiation with you. You might need it in the future and your body can only tolerate a certain amount.'" I remembered, too, that he did not even recommend that my mastectomy be followed by reconstruction, and I agreed; I had been through too much surgery. Years later, when I raised the question with a feeble wisecrack ("How about some new boobs for me?"), he gave me the go-ahead. But by that time, it was I who did not want to risk silicone, or even saline water-filled, implants.

I had never met Dr. Alley before, but I thought she would be just the right person to talk with about the breast cancer scene as we neared the end of the century. Years ago when I had asked my competent Harvard- and NCI-trained Washington oncologist Philip Cohen which of the burgeoning number of local surgeons I should recommend to breast patients who called me, he suggested Dr. Kathy Alley. And I had seen her featured on the cover of the November 1993 *Washingtonian* magazine, where I read that she was "highly regarded for both surgical and communications skills."

"Sometimes I think I've sent you half your practice," I told her when I called for an appointment, "and I've never had any negative feedback." I could soon see why. Sitting in the waiting room, I watched this tall blond physician escort a mother and daughter from the back office area, a cheerful multicolored scarf softening her starched white coat. All three were chatting, and the patient, whom I estimated to be fiftyish, seemed comfortable and animated. "Just a second," said Dr. Alley. "I want to give you the name of another plastic surgeon so you'll have more choices." She left and returned with the name and another booklet to add to those in the patient's bag.

Had this smiling woman just been diagnosed with breast cancer? Disbelieving, I asked the question once I was seated across the desk from Kathy Alley. She nodded and indicated that this woman was no exception. She makes a habit, she told me, of explaining everything carefully to patients with the help of

illustrated booklets, outlining their options (but never, even
in answer to questions, their possibly depressing statistical
chances), drawing diagrams, writing down salient points.
"There is no advantage to a negative attitude, *ever*, with breast
cancer patients. Especially at the beginning of treatment, they
need a positive outlook, so I am positive. I don't think you
should mislead people, but geez, any of us could be hit by a
truck walking down the street tomorrow."

A great deal had changed, the surgeon agreed, in the twenty-
three years since my first mastectomy, and since she graduated
from medical school in 1979. To start with, the "one-stage operation," which had been such a problem for me early on, might
still be performed by some doctors, but "it's unusual. There's
no reason to do it."

Biopsies, she explained, are almost all done under local anesthesia with sedation, and some simple ones with just local
anesthesia: "There's no reason to put people to sleep." The incidence of breast cancer has increased (15 percent since 1975). But
there are more early diagnoses than there used to be, probably
because of improvements in mammography. And more intra-
ductal or noninvasive cancers—about twice the number of the
biopsies found when she was in training.

Better mammography and greatly increased public conscious-
ness of the disease have, of course, played a role in bringing
patients to the doctor earlier. And patient fear has eased in
many ways; there is less to be fearful about. After the biopsy—
which includes estrogen and progesterone receptor tests to tell
whether hormones affect the way a cancer grows (only guessed
at, in my case)—Dr. Alley sees almost all her patients within
twenty-four hours to go over their pathology reports and explain
their options.

And, of course, surgeons (including plastic surgeons) and their
oncologist colleagues have more to offer. Though there are still
patients who are not candidates for breast preservation (usually
because their "multifocal" tumors are found in multiple spots
in the same breast), most are. "In my practice," said Dr. Alley,
"between 80 and 85 percent choose lumpectomy with axillary
[node] dissections and radiation [without which there is a

25–40 percent chance of recurrence]; the others, mastectomy with reconstruction, though I know the statistics vary in different parts of the country."

According to an article published in the March 1998 issue of the *Journal of the American College of Surgeons*, large population studies tell a different story: nationwide, more than 50 percent of early-stage breast cancer patients—those most likely to be eligible for breast-conserving therapy (BCT)—continue to undergo mastectomy. This despite the fact that medical contraindications of BCT were not found to be a major factor in high mastectomy rates and that, given a choice, 81 percent of eligible patients chose BCT, independent of age or race. (For more on age-related bias, see chapter 5.)

As I listened to Dr. Alley, I could almost taste my feelings—joy at the progress being made but a bit of envy at the manifold options offered more and more women. Spurning the controversial silicone and even the now popular saline implants, more of her middle-aged patients are turning, said the breast surgeon, to the newer "in" reconstructive procedure, the "TRAM" flap (wherein doctors take muscle from the abdomen—as in a "tummy tuck"—and make a breast out of it) and the less often used dorsal flap (wherein they take the muscle from the back). But such operations are likely to be rejected by older women because they involve such major surgery and by younger ones because they prefer implants, which involve less scarring as well as less invasive surgery.

The latest national figures from the Plastic Surgery Information Service tell a similar story: of the some fifty thousand women choosing breast reconstruction in 1997, close to a quarter chose the TRAM flap operation (and a smaller proportion, flaps using skin from other parts of the body), while the rest chose some type of implant. A whopping 74 percent of those with implants opted for saline-water-filled implants, whereas only roughly 12 percent chose gel-filled. I was glad to know this; even though many respected scientists have given the use of silicone gel in breast implants the OK so far as serious disease consequences are concerned, I have been wary of silicone implants ever since this thick substance made me shiver as it leaked from my first artificial breast (which I dubbed my "explant") onto my skin years ago.

Importantly, oncologists are using adjuvant chemotherapy more and more frequently. "When I was in training," Dr. Alley continued, "you did not get chemotherapy unless you had three or more positive lymph nodes." Now, she continued, women with positive lymph nodes and premenopausal women with lesions one centimeter or larger are included. (And an NCI consensus conference has suggested that adjuvant therapy of some type—whether it be chemotherapy or tamoxifen—be given all women with node-positive invasive cancers or those with negative nodes but tumors larger than one centimeter.)

I looked at her a bit wistfully. "I really feel I would have done much better," I said, "if that sort of adjuvant therapy had been available to me. I might not even have had metastases. Cancer is such a sneaky disease—"

"It is a sneaky disease. But it's important for women to realize that even if the cancer spreads and they develop metastatic disease, that does not mean they're going to die of it. Look at you!"

I did look at me and tried to remember my mother's admonition that you have to live in your own time as Dr. Alley went on to describe other therapies still being studied for women at high risk for metastases: "Transplants, for instance. They harvest out what are called stem cells from your blood—they no longer have to go into your bones for marrow—and save them while they give you strong chemo to kill the cancer cells; then they give you back your own healthy cells."

Would she have such an experimental procedure herself? "My feeling is if I had breast cancer and knew I was in an extremely high risk group for recurrence, I would do whatever I thought possible to reduce my risks, including transplantation. We don't really know yet about long-range effects of transplants, but they're beginning to show some benefit. So a transplant would, at the most, help me and, at the least, buy me time. After all, who knows what they will come up with within the next five years?"

The surgeon, I assumed, was thinking of all the other promising new treatments under study: Monoclonal antibodies such as

Herceptin (which slows cancer activity in certain patients).
Growth factors that increase the production of blood cells to
replace those destroyed by chemotherapy. New uses of the hormonal drugs tamoxifen and raloxifene (approved by the Food
and Drug Administration for halting bone loss, this drug shares
tamoxifen's potential for preventing breast cancer without triggering other malignancies). Drugs—thus far successful only in
mice—that will destroy the blood vessels feeding tumors and so
strangle them. And farther down the pike, some sort of genetic
therapy.

Such a plethora of options, no matter how hopeful, can carry a
price tag. Of course, some survivors sail through all the decision
making and treatment, if not happily, at least smoothly, and
with a minimum of trauma. My friend Louisa, a social worker,
considered herself "a lucky woman" to have a gynecologist who
insisted on sending her for a mammogram because of a suspicious thickening in her breast.

After diagnosis, she moved ahead competently and optimisti-
cally, step by step, "not particularly frightened," identifying an
oncologist, deciding on the lumpectomy with axillary dissec-
tion (nodes negative), scheduling the ensuing course of radiation
at Cape Cod Hospital so she could get on with her summer vacation ("Natalie, without radiation, there's a 34 percent chance
of recurrence and that's too great! And it would have been
depressing to turn our vacation upside down to sit around in
Washington while I was radiated.") Still, she could remember
two disturbing times: first, when the Cape Cod doctors suggested she postpone her radiation until she got home (her
Washington internist and oncologist were "horrified" at the
suggestion, and she turned it down flat); second, the fright she
felt when she was first left absolutely alone with a giant
machine shooting radiation at her, in touch with the world
only by microphone.

But the truth is that not even the most exalted and seemingly
invincible people among us are exempt from the shaking up cancer can give you, in a medical world that has so much more, now,
to offer than it had when I was first diagnosed. When I intro-

duced Justice Sandra Day O'Connor to the National Coalition for Cancer Survivorship Assembly in 1994, I did not know quite what to expect. The first woman to serve on the Supreme Court, this reserved legal virtuoso, a very private person, had not spoken publicly about her breast cancer experience before.

Her speech, carried to the nation through the miracle of television, electrified all of us survivors in the hall and elsewhere. Confessing that she was "quite unprepared" for the suddenness and the urgency of the rapid treatment decisions to be made and for the way even the word *cancer* overwhelms the psyche, she told how "everything had to stop" while she focused on her options: "A very tough time."

Before, she had thought that if she got sick, the doctor said what ought to be done, and that was the end of it. "Right? Wrong! . . . You run into this whole business of what do you do, a lumpectomy, a mastectomy or a radiation approach, do you have chemotherapy, do you not, if you have surgery what kind, how extensive." Though she had friends to consult and her husband came with her to meet her doctors, they were strangers to medical terms, and it was "like cramming for an exam in college."

In the end, she proceeded the way she did in Court: she tried to learn everything she could about her case, do as much research as possible, and then make her decision. "I don't look back," she said. Her decision was to have the mastectomy, but she confessed to finding the postoperative period depressing; she felt weak, emotional, and in some discomfort, and all this was hard on her family. Gradually, she began to edge her way back into her work and even onto the golf course and tennis court.

Justice O'Connor told us of her dream: "To have all those tests done, the biopsies and the X rays and whatever it is they are going to do, get all the information, and then have a consultation with all the experts available at the same time . . . to help you reach a decision." Moving from specialist to specialist— surgeon, radiologist, oncologist, plastic surgeon—and relying on the care of doctors, nurses, and psychologists, with "separate appointments and separate approaches [with] one doctor not hearing what the other said, increased the uncertainty and increased the trauma."

Listening to her, I thought, if health professionals at a top-notch treatment facility cannot provide this sort of cohesive service for a VIP justice, they certainly would not do it for us ordinary mortals.

But I was proved wrong. The Lombardi Cancer Center at Georgetown University Medical Center did make O'Connor's dream come true for other patients. Nowadays, a breast cancer consultative group composed of a medical oncologist, radiation oncologist, breast surgeon, and psychologist (a team coordinated by a nurse-clinician) meets together one morning a week with between one and four newly diagnosed patients and their partners (or significant others) to go over their individual cases, discuss and take questions about recommended options, and help them make difficult choices. Patients are encouraged to tape the proceedings.

What a wonderful innovation! Even when this sort of breaking out of the mold does not occur, or in cases in which it is not necessary, it helps when even one of your doctors takes the time to relate to you when you are dealing with cancer news, bad and good. At the end of my interview with Dr. Alley, I thanked her for her time, and for her willingness, not only to talk to me but to listen and ponder my questions. Had she always responded to people that way?

"I think I got part of that from my mother," she replied. My mother was a nurse in Oklahoma—a wonderful nurse—so it comes naturally, and I've acquired more skills over the years." As for time, she feels "you have to make time for people. Everyone you talk to has different needs. One person says, 'all right, it's obvious, I had already decided on that, where do we go from here?' Another says 'I'd like you to explain this or what about that.' But if you're not willing to take the time to spend with a patient, you shouldn't be in medicine."

Amen. We survivors need time to talk and listen and absorb information and consider our options. We need time to build up hope. For without hope, we do not flourish.

3 ❧ Talking and Hoping

"We're talking about how we relate to doctors," Group leader Sally Jo explained as Alicia took her place at the table. "Sometimes I think I spend all my time picking up after doctors."

"I left my cold as ice oncologist early on when he told me he had little hope for me; the odds were against me," Megan said. "He didn't even say 'I might be wrong, but. . . .' I switched to a new doctor. She said, 'Only the Lord can predict your odds.'"

"Your first oncologist couldn't have had very good lines to the Almighty," the social worker observed. "You look as though you're going to outlive us all, Megan."

Lester seemed paler, thinner than last summer. "My doctor," he said, looking to his wife Lucy for support. "He takes care. Busy, though. So many patients."

Lucy, a stout woman with a habit of pulling her mouth down when she tensed up, said Lester's doctor usually answered all their questions. Megan thought that highly unusual. She talked about the innate empathetic nature of women health professionals. Alicia remembered Dr. McBride's nurse, who seemed only slightly more aware than he of how crucial to a patient's spirits can be getting the results of a scan before, instead of after a weekend.

"Maybe health professionals are not well enough trained to pay attention to their patients' feelings," she ventured.

Mark talked glibly. He thought that medical students were so overworked and had so much highly complex scientific material to master that they did not have time to learn about human problems like fear of recurrence.

"What can we do to make our caregivers more responsive to our emotional needs?" Sally Jo asked.

Megan thought patients have to learn to be more assertive with their doctors. Isabelle agreed, but pointed out some don't want to participate in decision making as much as others: when her doctor coolly laid out her breast surgery options, then sent her home to decide for herself whether a lumpectomy or mastectomy would be better, she had anguished so long that her husband proposed a "Honk if you think I should have a lumpectomy" bumper sticker!

Laughter. Then silence in the hospital meeting room. The Group sat, safe, relaxed; they knew a measure of hope.

> —Natalie Davis Spingarn,
> *Background Music*
> (a novel in progress)

Survivors, of course, differ. Thirsting for facts about our disease, some run to the library or bookstore to bone up on it; others want the barest minimum. But most of us crave some time to discuss new, mysterious, and often threatening facts about our bodies and minds with our doctors and ask questions about what we're told. Our need for this information, and beyond that, our sensitivity to the way it is conveyed, change as we acquire more experience as survivors.

Surveyed at the end of 1996, an international group of patients and their supporters I have worked with as a member of *The Patient's Network* editorial board agreed, hands-down, that over time, both patients' information needs and their ability to satisfy them change. So does their level of sophistication and their state of "readiness to learn."

My innocence of the problems surrounding patient-doctor communications at the beginning of my cancer journey astounds me now. Back then, I questioned little; I accepted gratefully the way my surgeon, in the quiet privacy of his office, told me matter-of-factly that the hard lump in my breast needed exploring. Later, when he sat down in my hospital room, still in his green surgical suit, and reported that he had removed my breast because the lump was malignant, I listened once again with quiet relief. It was "garden variety," he said, small but *there.*

He thought my chances were good because he had "gotten it all." Some time afterward the late Harvard Medical School psychiatrist and coping authority Dr. Avery Weisman told me that what he and other surgeons really mean by "getting it all" is "as much out as possible, there may be more."

While my surgeon spoke, I listened numbly. The pain flooded my torn chest as I absorbed the news. It did not occur to me to press him about my chances, or about the number of nodes he had extracted from my armpit, or indeed about the fact that, over the decade I had been his patient, although I had had regular examinations, he ordered none of the mammograms then beginning to be used (because, he told me, of my dense breasts).

When he left the room, I wept for my lost breast. But I trusted this surgeon, skilled at dealing with patients as well as cutting their bodies; his sense of optimism rubbed off on me. His rosy prognosis agreed with me, and I believed it. What if I had not? What if my doctor had conveyed hopelessness instead of hope?

I think I would have despaired. I would have been ten times more vulnerable to the hopeless remarks by doctors that many hear, such as, "I've seen this go pretty fast," or (to another woman), "You won't die of this stomach cancer. But it's already spread here—see this X ray?—to the liver." I would have been desolate instead of just appalled by the resident who bade me a postmastectomy farewell—a farewell that triggered my suspicion that modern doctor-patient communications needed reexamination.

I was sitting on a bench near a hospital nursing station, waiting to be dismissed, when this resident approached with a polite: "How are you?"

"Okay." And then, because that did not seem enough, "I get blue once in a while, but that's all. The doctors tell me a little postoperative weeping is par for the course."

"Ah," he answered. "You like to read, don't you?" He had observed the books and magazines on my bed.

"Yes."

"Well, you should read *On Death and Dying.*"

Having consigned me to the grave, he allowed that the operation I had was often successful. Then he disallowed such optimism by going through Elisabeth Kübler-Ross's thesis: at first the dying person denies his or her situation, then feels angry,

asking, "Why me?" Before he could develop it further through
the bargaining, depression, and acceptance stages, my son
grabbed my arm and steered me away.

Back home, I began to think about his heart-wrenching
approach. As I went through unwelcome and unexpected metastases, my involvement with my doctors deepened, and so did my
interest in patient-doctor communications. I began to observe
the way various doctors talked to me and my fellow survivors
and to talk with seasoned experts about the potentially stunning
power of a doctor's words.

What I learned was that while changes in medical technology
and procedure were subject to serious scientific trial and experi-
mentation, others, especially changes in medical attitudes,
often were not. For example, 90 percent of the doctors responding to a questionnaire in 1961 said they preferred not to tell cancer patients their diagnoses. In 1977, the same questionnaire
showed a complete reversal: 97 percent of those responding said
it was their general policy to tell patients the truth. As medical
science has acquired more to offer survivors, this is still probably the case in the United States, though "truth" is told with
varying degrees of skill and empathy.

The team reporting this policy turnabout in the *Journal of the
American Medical Association* (JAMA) deplored the fact that in
the late seventies, as sixteen years earlier, "physicians were bas-
ing their policies on emotion-laden personal convictions,"
rather than on scientific studies of the effect on patients of what
they say.

Covering the American Psychiatric Association meeting in
the spring of 1978, I breakfasted with Dr. Edward Gottheil, who
had led a Philadelphia medical team in doing such a study. Comparing recently hospitalized cancer patients who were not aware
of their diagnoses with similar patients who were so aware, the
team concluded that because awareness may be beneficial for
some but not for all terminally ill patients, caution and judg-
ment should be exercised in sharing information with them.

Though this was a surprising finding for that time, it did not
surprise Dr. Gottheil. After all, he asked, was not the word *cancer* often equated with death, and the knowledge of impending

death once part of punishment meted out for criminal behavior? Had not Dostoyevsky been emotionally scarred for life when he was marched into the prison courtyard and prepared to be "shot"? Dr. Gottheil himself, he reported, had seen increasing numbers of psychiatric referrals among "informed patients." The knowledge of impending death, he had found, was attended by fear and depression as often as by courage and dignity.

I listened, intrigued, and wondered. My own heart had felt mighty heavy after doctor remarks like "I've seen this go pretty fast" or "Obviously the operation did not have the expected results. I hope there's something we can do for you." Or even, "Well, would you like to live forever?" I could empathize with the Syrian king who, the Bible tells us, sent a messenger to Elisha to ask whether he would survive his sickness. The prophet responded, "Go, say unto him: 'Thou shall surely recover'; howbeit the Lord hath shown me that he shall surely die."

I agreed: hopefulness should be maintained at almost all costs, not so much by selectively withholding information but by presenting it in an encouraging, positive way. Still, as a modern person, I knew I certainly did not want to be kept in the dark about the fact that I had cancer (and even if I had been so inclined, it would have been impossible if I wanted to be treated at a proud, expert cancer center). As my old friend and college contemporary Dr. Betty Hamburg, a skillful psychiatrist and professor at Mount Sinai School of Medicine, put it: "It's scary to know. But it's also scary not to know."

1982. By the time of my second breast tumor, I had come to realize that it was not so much exactly what a doctor told me that was important but how he or she conveyed the message about the increasing number of options open to me. I also had come to understand that some physicians simply understand better than others that stressed patients, confronted by confusing, contradictory medical predictions and choices, can have trouble absorbing abstract concepts no matter what their education or degree of sophistication. Blotting out everything else, they tend to focus on what Betty Hamburg calls key "buzzwords" (like "life expectancy," "guarded prognosis," or "complications"). As the likelihood of information overload increases, it takes greater skill to strike the fine balance between informing patients when necessary and burdening them with unnecessary, perhaps harmful details—often while we sit or lie vulnerable on the examination table, our faded examination robes held together by frayed strings.

Doctors skilled in the art as well as the science of medicine respond more sensitively to survivors' individual sensibilities— their different backgrounds, different tolerance for pain, different resources and family situations, as well as different attitudes and beliefs about this world, and for some, the next. Never, for example, did I feel depressed when I left Tom Fahey's office at Sloan-Kettering, no matter what bad news he had to impart. He always explained carefully what was going on in my body, in a nonthreatening way. He could say the worst things without leaving me decimated. Thus I had a "crummy," not a "horrible," disease, or should my tumor "start to cook again," not, "should your tumor metastasize to the liver." When I asked him, "How can you stand dealing with this awful disease every day?" he answered that "nice patients" like me help him do his job. Such a remark helps make you a partner in a difficult but controllable enterprise.

I know that not everyone's experience at this distinguished cancer center has been as positive as mine; indeed, the staff seems the first to admit when things go wrong and to try to make amends. And I know that survivors have found talented oncologist/communicators in many hospitals and treatment centers. Still, not only has the staff at Sloan-Kettering treated me successfully, but, importantly, they have usually made me feel that something could be done to alleviate my pain, perhaps even to curb my cancer. Most have understood the clues we survivors invariably give as to what we want to know. These may be silent: we can just look away, avoid eye contact, or stay quiet (*Enough*). Or we can head for the library or World Wide Web and inform the doctor of what we found (*More*). Other cues are spoken: "My sister's doctor told her exactly what's what and she's off to the Caribbean" (*Please tell me exactly what's what*), or "I'm paying you to worry about it; I don't want to worry about it" (*Enough!*).

Importantly, too, Dr. Fahey, my anchor at Sloan-Kettering, has never hurled statistics about my chances for survival at me. He did this as a young specialist, he once told me, but stopped when experience proved to him that patients are human beings—each different from the other—not statistics on a curve. This realization came after a patient he counseled to "get her affairs in order," because of her dim statistical outlook, turned up flying an airplane some years later, while her daughter, anticipating her mother's death, had landed in deep psychotherapy.

A landmark telephone call from my Washington oncologist crystallized my views about patient-doctor communications. For some weeks, the pathologists had been testing a suspicious lump in my remaining breast; in the face of conflicting evidence, they had a difficult diagnosis to make.

Now, the doctor socked it to me. The lump had proved cancerous. Believing it probably had metastasized from my other breast, he had an opinion: "You have one year to live," he told me, "maybe two."

After eight years of survivorship, I simply could not handle this cruel news. Distraught, I rushed up to New York. "Who told him how long you have?" asked Tom Fahey. "How does he know?" Indeed, it turned out he did not know. The cancer proved to be a new primary, not a metastasis, and I am still alive more than fifteen years later. But I had a new mission: teasing out the elements of effective patient-doctor communications and trying, in turn, to communicate them to patients and young doctors alike, wherever they may live and work.

I proceeded in different ways. As a journalist, I challenged doctors who tended to blame patients for any breakdown in communication and burden us with unnecessary gory disease details even while telling us to adopt a feisty hopeful attitude and lead a quality life (the headline on the "Second Opinion" column I wrote for the *Washington Post* read: "Give It to Me Straight, Doc, but with Sensitivity").

And I embarked on a project in an area new to me: film. On a press club trip to Finland, I sat with a fellow traveler on a rocky hillside near the Arctic Circle watching a lonely reindeer graze.

"Considering all you've been through—all that cancer," this Public Broadcasting Service executive observed, "you certainly get around." She encouraged me to submit an outline to PBS for a show on a cancer survivor's problems and challenges.

The resulting film, "A Different Kind of Life," aired as part of Jim Lehrer's *U.S. Chronicle* series. Along with a teenager who had lost her leg to cancer (rarely seen anymore, so skilled have surgeons become at substituting healthy for cancerous bone sections) and a young forest ranger–bride with Hodgkin's disease, I helped dramatize the good and less good news that though more people were living longer with cancer, they often have to live a different kind of life. Directed by virtuoso producer Ricki Green, the film showed survivors working hard and playing happily, though they still often had to continue in heavy, or at least pesky, medical treatment, wear wigs and prostheses, and pace themselves carefully.

Working on the film expanded my horizons, as well as those—I hope—of its large audience. As a writer, I had long been acquainted with the old saying that a picture is worth a thousand words. Now I was sure of it—and I thoroughly enjoyed working, not alone at the computer, but out in the mainstream along with a bunch of talented people—and then seeing immediate results. So I took my mission a step further and asked Ricki if she would work with me (along with a younger producer, Jill Clevinger) on a new project—an educational videotape on patient-doctor communications that could be used both by patients and medical caregivers. When Ricki agreed, I set about seeking funding (from the American Cancer Society, and later, the Picker Foundation), securing administrative support (from the National Health Policy Forum), lining up a cast, and finally writing a "treatment" for the script.

As *Patients and Doctors: Communication Is a Two-Way Street* opens, Sloan-Kettering psychiatry chief Dr. Jimmie Holland (a member of our film advisory committee) counsels Carol Levine, a breast cancer survivor. Carol had been getting along nicely with her doctor team when she suffered some unusual bleeding that forced her to go to an unfamiliar gynecologist.

Without looking at her medical records or examining her or asking any further questions, a shocked Carol tells Dr. Holland, the new gynecologist simply stated: "Oh well, you probably have another malignancy. . . . You'll have to have a D&C right away."

"I really felt unable to even hear it," Carol said. "I was mad. I said no, I'm not having anything right away. I'm putting on my clothes and going home and I can't talk to you anymore. I really was just devastated."

Such experiences, Dr. Holland tells her patient, are "unfortunately not rare, because bloopers happen. People speak thoughtlessly without realizing the impact that it has upon an individual who is frightened, worried, and listening for likely the most negative things."

Other patients report their reactions to similar "bloopers." In a group led by social worker Mary Ellen Bowles, several women tell of their distress when, like me, they had gotten bad news over the telephone. Another explains the painful effect of as small a nuance as a consulting dermatologist's telling her, "So you're in remission," when she had thought herself cancer-free.

Family as well as patient can be affected, Vee Burke remembers. She and her husband were on an emotional roller coaster when he fell ill with pancreatic cancer. Questioning him coldly about his history in the hospital, a young intern or resident asked, "What was your profession?" She stared at this robust young doctor for a minute, then responded: "What *is* his profession?"

He stared back: "Well you *are* an optimist." This seemed untenable to Vee. "We were no optimists. We knew that our days were numbered, but we were struggling together, living together, loving together, working together, and clinging to a little hope." Health caregivers as well as patients in this film speak of the necessity for new roles: for doctors to act more as coaches—always honest but careful of their language, kind, tactful, and hopeful—and for patients and those who love them to speak up. Or, as one put it, to "be a bit more important in the whole thing."

Barrie Cassileth, Ph.D., then a psychologist at the University of Pennsylvania Medical School (also a member of our *Patients and Doctors* advisory committee), took up this theme and gave

the film its name. Communication, she points out, is a two-way
street; it is a patient's responsibility to tell the physician outright or give the physician cues about the amount of information
he or she would like to have. Above all, she urges patients not to
be afraid to ask "silly" questions, for "there is no such thing as a
stupid question."

Echoing her views, the physician-performers in the award-
winning film stress the "art" of caring for patients. At George
Washington University Medical School, Dr. Robert Siegal lis-
tens to a cue from a very ill patient that he was comfortable with
the doctor as primary decision maker: "You know best."

And at Sloan-Kettering, Tom Fahey serves as a role model to
busy medical students, warning that "one of the most important
things you can leave with a patient is that you've got time for
them: To stand by the doorstop or at the entrance to the patient's
room and look like you're ready to fly down the hall is just terribly disturbing to people."

The world of survivor and doctor has turned over many times
by century's end. In the course of a little more than a decade,
paternalism has given way to partnership. There seems to be
less physician patronization, less patient passivity, and more
involvement of both in decision making.

With more treatments to offer and more survivors asserting
their rights, Barrie Cassileth (now affiliated with Harvard,
Duke, and the University of North Carolina) points out that it
would be next to impossible not to be open about diagnoses or
explain options. In *Patients and Doctors,* she had explained to
medical students that they should always attach a treatment
plan to a diagnosis, saying, "Here is what we are going to do."
Now, she feels, a physician would say, "Here are your options.
What would *you* like to do?"

At least one enlightened expert research team, Sheldon Green-
field, M.D., and Sherrie Kaplan, Ph.D, had shown that faulty
communication can affect more than survivors' feelings; it can
affect their doctors' ability to treat them and consequently their
health. In a multitude of studies reported in professional journals, these two senior scientists at the New England Medical

Center have demonstrated that patient passivity during office visits relates negatively to health status in a number of diseases (including breast cancer). And vice versa: the more questions patients ask, the more interruptions and statements they make, the more "controlling" they are—the more their physiologic health improves and the less limited is their function.

The lesson of this research—that patients should speak up and back to doctors, and conversely, that doctors should encourage them to do so—was certainly not lost on me. With a decade's experience in the survivorship movement under my belt (as both an editor and an officer of the National Coalition for Cancer Survivorship), I had become a stronger, more assertive survivor, able to "titrate" information—which means, in medicine, put in a little of this and a little of that, until you achieve a comfortable balance. I could ask a medical student doing a rotation in my internist's office if he minded my telling him something; when he nodded OK, I advised him not to look at his watch repeatedly while he was dealing with patients. "I know you're busy," I said, "but you're going out into a competitive marketplace, and patients don't like consulting doctors who send them a trivializing message."

I well realize that knowledge is power. But I am able to seek information and speak up when I need to—telling my excellent, charming, and usually empathetic (but terribly busy) head and neck surgeon, for example, that though I appreciated his calling me to see how I felt the night before surgery to excise a squamous cancer from my tongue, I was distressed when he called me "Nancy."

"My name," I told him, "is Natalie." More important, when he approached me with preoperative consent forms, I told him, "I don't want to wake up without a tongue." He answered that he was sure he would have to excise only a small piece.

"You were sure before the biopsy that the lesion was benign," I told him; "it turned out to be malignant."

And he said, "I hear you."

All in all, as Lombardi Cancer Center psychologist Julia Rowland explains, there has been a general increase in doctor sensitivity to survivor psychosocial concerns; most doctors, for

example, had "stopped beating up on patients with statistics."
And on the other end of the two-way street, the number of
patients seeking "holistically" minded doctors and therapies
considered warm, understanding, and patient-friendly (as we
will see later in this book) has surely soared. One even hears
stories of oncologists who pray for and with their patients; I
have not experienced this! But in July 1998 I noted a story in the
New York Times illustrated by a photo of the Dalai Lama, his
palms pressed together in prayer, leaning over a doctor role-play-
ing a patient at a New York City hospital teaching conference.

Yet several factors continue to work against optimal communications between doctor and patient. For one thing, though the
importance of rapport between the two is generally recognized,
young doctors are still probably not being adequately trained in
how to build it. The American Medical Association reported
that, of the 125 United States medical schools, only 11 required
their students to take separate courses in communication skills
in 1996–97. Although an additional 14 offered separate elective
courses, and although most said they covered communication
skills as part of regular courses, there was no consistent rein-
forcement of these skills throughout medical training. And the
amount of "hard" material students must master left little time
and energy for what weary medical students dub "soft stuff."
Though some lucked onto role models they could emulate,
others did not.

What's more, the era of managed care has left many physicians in a position wherein they simply cannot communicate
with their patients effectively. Third, fourth, and sometimes, it
seems, even fifth parties like insurance or managed care companies often restrict what doctors can and cannot do, even the
amount of time spent with patients and also the amount of dis-
closable information not under "gag rule." Both doctor and
patient can be left dissatisfied and uncomfortable with the
resulting dialogue.

"'Hope' is the thing with feathers— / That perches in the soul—,"
wrote Emily Dickinson. Hope has certainly perched upon my
soul in my years of survivorship. And I have come to see that

poor communication can affect even more than just which treatments and medications doctors prescribe. It can affect a vital, if elusive, sentiment even the most accomplished poets have found difficult to define but one that the eminent psychiatrist Karl Menninger called a part of being human.

Looking back over what I have said and written during my cancer journey, again and again I find myself alluding to my need to reinforce the hope that sustains my life. As I wrote in *Parade* magazine in the early 1980s, "It helps most of all if you stay near people and things that give you hope and away from whatever takes it away"—near people who encourage you to keep fighting and, conversely, away from anyone who tells you long, sad stories about how you're going to die on Thursday. "If I listen to them," I confessed, "I *will* die on Thursday."

In other words, we survivors need hope in order to deal—to cope—with the roller coaster of survivorship. At one time, I confess, I did not cotton to the overworked word *cope*, a holdover from my days as an assistant to Connecticut's Senator Abraham Ribicoff. ("Don't use *cope*," he once told me. "People who sit on the floor say *cope*.") But now I know no other word that will fit the bill. It seems to point the way toward what the late psychiatrist Dr. Avery Weisman, in his fine booklet *Coping with Cancer*, called "safe conduct": conducting survivors, and helping them to conduct themselves, through the hanging-in maze of problems and fears—a dimension beyond diagnosis, treatment, and relief.

Weisman, a professor of psychiatry at Harvard Medical School who directed the Omega research project at Massachusetts General Hospital, explained that the coping process combines several different kinds of strategies. These are both active and passive, depending on the purpose, and vary from seeking more information (*rational inquiry*) and sharing concern and talk with others (*mutuality*) to trying to forget, putting your dilemma out of your mind (*suppression*), or blaming someone or something else (*externalize, project*). No strategy works for all of your problems, whether it be laughing it off (*affect reversal*) or doing other things for distraction (*displacement/redirection*).

Some work better and more often than others. Denial, which revises or reinterprets a portion of the painful reality you face, can be part of the coping process. It is, as one doctor put it, the "morphine of the soul." If it is not used excessively—to avoid necessary diagnosis and treatment, for instance, or to avoid dealing with unfinished business—it can help survivors avoid what threatens in the future and hold fast to what is helpful in the past.

How you define hope will give you clues to achieving it. From the psychiatric literature I found that hope is a learned response, produced by optimism, expectation, and recollection of past successes and failures augmented by supportive and successful examples. If hope can be learned, then it seemed to me both that caregivers should strive constantly and painstakingly to teach it and that survivors should try to use it.

The need for hope is complex and can be expressed by many different kinds of people in different ways, at different times in their journeys. "Miracles do happen," a very sick hospital roommate told me; "maybe one will happen to me." I do not know if it did. But it could have; there are no fast rules. A seasoned internist told me once that every experienced physician has seen an established cancer simply vanish. Extremely rare, but it happens. Why take away our hope when we may be among the lucky ones?

Besides, as many survivors have suspected and several scholars have pointed out in the past, just as hope sustains life, hopelessness can cause death. In his book *Hope,* for example, psychosomaticist Dr. Arnold Hutschnecker reported many cases of the power of active hope—"an inner mental force," triggering the human will and mobilizing vast individual energies to overcome obstacles.

Patients fight cancer, Hutschnecker explained, with hope—hope of a cure, hope of a chance to live longer. He cited a study of two hundred patients, reporting that people without hope see no end to their suffering but those with hope have confidence in the desirability of survival. Indeed, when death nears—and it is by no means always immediate, even in "incurable" cases—patients can continue to be active, working and participating in social activities. With the focus on comfort and pain control, the bare possibility of one chance in one thousand of surviving can help patients psychologically endure what might otherwise be intolerable.

Another expert, Johns Hopkins professor emeritus Dr. Jerome Frank, reported that in civilized as well as primitive societies, a person's conviction that his or her predicament is hopeless may cause or hasten disintegration and death. Why else is the death of aged people shortly after admission to state mental hospitals unduly high? What other reason than hopelessness, aggravated by abandonment, for the fact that no adequate cause of death is found at the time of autopsy?

Writing in a scientific paper, Dr. Frank told about the striking results of a rehabilitation team who went into a chronic disease hospital that had previously warehoused "hopeless" patients with a program designed to change the atmosphere and give them hope that they could get better and get out into the community: some 70 percent of the patients who had been hospitalized three to ten years left the hospital; 40 percent of them became self-supporting.

Such earlier research with cancer patients, according to Elizabeth J. Clark, Ph.D., a medical sociologist and now president of the National Coalition for Cancer Survivorship (NCCS), focused on hopelessness. Perhaps, says Clark, whose interest in hope and communications led to an NCCS booklet called *Words That Heal, Words That Harm,* this is because a diagnosis of cancer used to be associated with certain death; hopelessness and an often restrictive helplessness naturally ensued.

She remembers a young surgeon who felt close to a patient of exactly the same age, with the same number of children. When the surgeon told his patient that his cancer had metastasized, the patient asked, "How bad is it?" (a question I have sometimes asked when I did not really want to know the answer—if it proved to be negative). The doctor answered, "If you have anything to do, you should go home and do it." Beset by tremendous anxiety, the patient went home and died six weeks later, of a heart attack.

Clark wonders why, as a frontier nation, a forward-looking nation with a future outlook almost ingrained in our beings, we Americans have found hope such a nebulous concept. Survivors without hope, without a glimmer of light at the end of the tunnel, she emphasizes, can become very discouraged and see no reason to accept or continue treatment—or even to pay attention to potentially valuable issues like nutrition. Still, hope has not been well studied.

Now that is changing; researchers are looking at hope as a measurable concept. In another NCCS booklet, *You Have the Right to Be Hopeful*, Clark pulls together some of what the recent hope literature tells us: it helps to know what hope does *not* mean. Hope is not *wishing*. We usually wish for something specific—to be a movie star, to be president. Such a wish is positive, but it is passive in nature and seldom based on reality. Nor is hope *optimism*, also a positive concept but one that does not necessarily give you a clear place to go. We all like to be around optimistic people, but we can get annoyed with Pollyannas who see only the good side of things. Besides, such blind optimism may close off painful feelings and result in inflexibility.

Wishing and optimism—both components of hope—have their place in our lives. But to live with cancer, to get through rigorous treatment, navigate the health care system, to fend off society's often negative views about the disease as a death sentence, you have to have a larger sense—a stronger hope experts have defined in different ways. I like psychologist C. R. Snyder's concept that such a hope combines *willpower*, the driving force to hopeful thinking, the mental energy that moves you toward a goal, with *waypower*, the mental capacity to find a way to reach these goals.

Pointing out that hope, as a way of thinking, feeling, and acting—in fact a prerequisite for action—is flexible and remains open to various possibilities, Clark argues that it is not a static concept. It changes, as reality changes; it has been called a "changing mosaic." So, new survivors usually enjoy therapeutic hope for a cure; later this may shift into hope for long-term control of your disease, or even for extended periods between recurrences.

And, still later, when survivorship stretches or when thera- peutic hope must be put aside, many find new hope in new achievements and new goals. In the past, I hoped to see my chil- dren "settled" and my grandchildren born. Now I hope to get this book (and perhaps others) written. I hope for a dignified death. And sometimes, like many of my survivor colleagues, when I dream of seeing my sister or mother again, I embrace a spiritual hope—even if my intellect tells me it is not based on pragmatic evidence. Hope, it seems, can transcend reality.

Led by nursing experts like Carol Farran and Mary Nowotny, researchers have started to map the hope landscape. They are formulating instruments whereby they can assess the amount of hope their patients harbor and so arrive at ways to help them. The Baylor University School of Nursing's Professor Nowotny, for one, suggests that a patient's hope be rated according to his or her *confidence in the outcome; relationships with others; possibility of a future; spiritual beliefs; active involvement;* and *inner readiness.*

If discouraged or unmotivated patients rate low on this last measurement, for instance, Professor Nowotny suggests several interventions. These include helping survivors identify and use existing strengths, encouraging them to keep a diary of feelings and experiences, and listening and staying with them.

Listen to them. Stay with them. And I would reemphasize, do not be put off if survivors seem to be harboring positive illusions —if they are, more technically, "in denial." Though denial gets a bum rap among many can-do Americans, it can be an important coping mechanism. As such, it can be of genuine help to those of us walking through thorny thickets.

I did not fully realize how useful were my impossible dreams until I wrote a piece headlined "Your Illusions May Be Good for You," based on research by a psychologist at the University of California at Los Angeles, Shelley Taylor. After intensively interviewing some seventy-eight breast cancer patients over a two-year period, Taylor concluded that people often allow themselves to use illusions in the face of threat and can even be "ultimately restored" by them—in the long as well as the short run.

Such persons, according to Taylor, use their illusions to search for the cause of their disease and often find positive implications in the results—no matter whether the "cause" they discover be true or false. They tilt at extraordinary windmills to control their disease, to prevent its return; again, it does not matter what they do—from meditation to adopting a healthy diet—it's the illusion that gives them some control. And they undertake a process of "self-enhancement"—restoring their self-image, protecting themselves by seeing themselves as more fortunate than others (a woman with a lumpectomy pitied those with a full mastectomy, another with a full mastectomy compared it to a double mastectomy, and so forth). If the illusion fails, they manufacture a new one—and find new ways of coping.

I was gratified to find evidence of what I had felt in my bones: my illusions about my survival and my ability to gain an upper hand over my disease, true or false, had motivated me to go out and do a great many things. Now it troubles me that some experts, particularly those working in the new, healthy effort to improve communications between doctors and dying patients, have become skeptical of illusions, pointing out that "false hope" has its own hazards, leading survivors to ignore present happenings while imagining positive future results.

For example, research conducted at Dana-Farber Cancer Institute and published in JAMA recently (a part of a larger continuing study of terminally ill patients, nationwide) reported that the majority of 917 hospitalized patients with advanced lung or colon cancer were far more optimistic than their doctors and that their optimism was often "misplaced" in that it caused them to choose useless, aggressive therapies that simply increased suffering and failed to prolong their lives.

But I am with the optimistic, hopeful patients in this study, whether or not they opted for aggressive treatment, who continued the good fight and so tried to savor the time left to them, each in his or her own way. And I wonder, with oncologist Dr. Thomas Smith, a faculty scholar with the Project on Death in America whose editorial accompanied the JAMA report, whether faulty doctor-patient communication (the withholding of information or its presentation in an unnecessarily harsh way) was at least somewhat at fault in those cases in which the patients or their families felt they had made the wrong choice.

Let us not forget that hope is a complicated, changing concept. Hope for many may still be therapeutic hope for a cure, or at least for a measure of control. So my hopes were recently raised by Dr. Michael Newman, the fine internist who now serves as my medical coach, helping me balance well-intentioned but at times overzealous specialist advice with my need to continue to live a quality life. When I called to tell him I was nervous about a forthcoming European trip because of implied medical pressure to stay put and have this skin cancer surgery or that testing and medication, his advice was brief: "Go to Europe. Send all of us [doctors] a postcard saying how much fun you're having."

Hope for others may be broader, involving things of the spirit as well as the body. And hope for all survivors labeled "terminally ill" should not be confused with hope for all cancer survivors at all times, in all situations. For me optimism—a part of hope—cannot be "misplaced"; imagining positive results in the future certainly does not preclude living as best we can in the here and now. In fact, it enhances our chances of doing so.

4 ❧ *Being Sick*
The Short Run

The hospital! Once you would have entered thinking it was a place to die in. You would have shuddered at the thought of it and all but abandoned hope when you were admitted. If you lived in Benjamin Franklin's time, that meticulous fellow's cornerstone inscription for Philadelphia's Pennsylvania Hospital was the best you could have said for it:

This Building
By the Bounty of the Government
And of Many Private Patients
Was Piously Founded
For the Relief of the Sick and Miserable
May the God of Mercies
Bless the Undertaking

Now, in an odd way, the hospital has come full circle. A decade or two ago, it had developed into a place to be born in and a place to be cured in, a haven during critical periods of your life that could last days or even weeks. You went there dreading the worst, but in your heart of hearts, you expected the wonderful. Medical progress gave you the chance to get not what you feared but what you hoped for, whether your illness turned out to be acute or chronic. And you got it in a bewilderingly new, high-tech, high-cost world unto itself.

Now the same high-tech hospital has become, as one physician I know put it, "nothing but an intensive care unit filled with very sick people." Its highly skilled staff still offers wondrous treatments, procedures, and so roads back to health. But for the cancer survivor, as for other chronically ill patients, hospitals have become only occasional, short-term havens—if they can be called havens at all.

With inpatient costs high and outpatient services used whenever possible, we survivors can no longer linger in a hospital bed for a week or two absorbing tender loving care and mobilizing strength after a tough medical encounter, as I did after my mastectomies in the 1970s and 1980s. You are out of that bed (and room) in a day or two at most; sometimes you have your operation before you ever reach it. "In-and-Out" or "Same Day Surgery" units are aptly named. And though "drive-through mastectomies" do not seem to be the order of the day, their occurrence has sparked demands for national legislation guaranteeing women at least forty-eight hours in the hospital following a mastectomy and produced similar laws in some fourteen states attempting to limit the "drive-through" phenomenon.

My own experience has shown me—if nothing else—the necessity for such mandates in this era of "dehospitalization." After many years as an outpatient, just when I thought I had kissed hospital beds good-bye for the duration, I had to have two small operations. For the first, an excision of a small squamous cancer of the tongue (1996), I arrived at 6:30 A.M. at New York City's Memorial Sloan-Kettering Cancer Center knowing I would be allowed to stay overnight only because I had developed a bleeding problem that demanded unusual postoperative attention.

I came much as the Lord had made me, without breakfast or anything but a sip of water, no makeup, no softening body lotion on my dry skin, no toilet water, no valuables, my husband clutching my overnight bag. With all pre-op tests done days before, I boarded a crowded elevator headed up to a holding room. Looking around at my elevator comrades, I empathized with those worried faces—after all, some were bound for far more extensive surgery than I. How long, I wondered, would they be allowed to stay in the hospital? If they were sent home, what

would they go home to? I smiled appreciatively at the elevator
operator when he sent us on our way with a prayer.

Soon I sat a bit nervously in a cubicle in a trusty faded hospital gown, having deposited my clothes and worldly goods with
my husband. When the gurney arrived, I was ready. Covered
with a warm blanket in the frigid operating room, I waited with
my surgeon for the bag of healthy platelets I might need if my
own did not perform correctly. I had time only for thankfulness
that I was in the hands of excellent physicians in a top-notch
cancer center that seemed prepared for the worst outcomes, as
well as the best, and managed a smile for the anesthesiologist. In
the end, I stayed in the hospital two nights and spent two more
uptown at my cousin Leigh's agreeable Riverside Drive apartment within a taxi ride of Sloan-Kettering's Urgent Care unit
(emergency room) until I could be checked and assured that
things had gone well and the danger of untoward bleeding had
passed.

For the second operation, a mundane hernia repair (1997),
arrangements had been made to admit me to Georgetown University Hospital in Washington, D.C., should it be absolutely
necessary. It was not; I arrived at the Same Day Surgery unit at
8:45 A.M. and left shortly after 2 P.M.—staggering but on two
feet, thinking that though I understood "their" need to keep
health costs down, I could never endure "same day" major cancer surgery. Even though I was not completely anesthetized or
"out" for this minor repair and never felt unsafe, I still felt
uncomfortable with the way I was pushed out of my recovery
cubicle after only a few hours, clutching my Tylenol tablets
and wondering how I could manage pain and possible side
effects at home. I imagined how difficult it must be to go home
the day of a mastectomy, with rubber tubes sticking out of my
body draining blood into a container, unable to move my arm
or go to the bathroom and afraid I might die or at least suffer
uncontrolled pain. (I strongly disagreed with a bigwig physician who told a "managed care" meeting I attended that
some patients preferred going home after surgery instead
of staying in the hospital overnight, and I told him so—
emphatically.)

All in all, then, such "dehospitalization," combined with the changing nature of cancer from a time-limited acute disease to a chronic illness that can last for years, has effectively limited our time as inpatients. Still, we survivors do spend some of our time in the hospital—most of it at the beginning of our hanging-in journeys. And even if you got the bad news in the doctor's office, hospital time often serves as the springboard for the survivorship experience and can set the tone for your approach to future care. As such, it is a significant part of the hanging-in life.

Survivors are often unprepared for what the social workers are pleased to call the "hospital ecology." I am reminded of this each time I pay a visit to a friend new to hospital life or even a fellow survivor with a recurrence. Sometimes, when I read a compelling account, like sportswriter Robert Lipsyte's often macho description of his own Sloan-Kettering stays, I am back again as a rookie survivor in what he calls the foreign "land of Malady," studying the chattering "up-tempo personalities" who do X rays and minor procedures and the other health care pros (whose power, however brief, "seems absolute") and wondering how I might protect my sense of vulnerability by asking questions in some unknown "right" way. And I can almost hear the "tumor humor" bandied about in room 831 by the author and his roommates, all members of the "young testicular set": the disease was different, but the bravado masking fear the same as that of the breast cancer patients floors above.

This state of unpreparedness still prevails. Like me, you have probably been in the hospital before only briefly to have babies (happily) or have your hemorrhoids repaired (a nuisance) or to visit a sick grandparent (a duty). Unless you considered yourself a very sophisticated consumer of hospital services—and we are getting more (though still not enough) of these feisty folks nowadays—you probably did not think long and hard about hospitals as part of a large industry, with managers trying to operate them as such.

And you probably did not shop carefully for a hospital, going to the library to check the accreditation status of community institutions or calling national hotlines to see whether a cancer center offering exactly what you needed was accessible to you.

Nor did you inquire as to whether a recommended hospital was affiliated with a medical school and had research and teaching obligations (and so good quality control). In the same way, you simply assumed your hospital had whatever expensive high-tech equipment you might need, as well as good lower-tech but all-important services (like respiratory or physical therapy) or an excellent nursing staff (both registered nurses and, importantly, non-RN aides) to take hands-on care of you.

What probably happened was that either your "fee for service" doctor stipulated one of the hospitals where he or she had "privileges," or your managed care plan offered you a limited choice of hospitals with which it is affiliated. Feeling apprehensive about what lay ahead—and perhaps physically ill as well—you may have agreed to whatever was suggested without much preliminary discussion at all. You wanted to hurry into the hospital and get that cancer out of you—the sooner the better.

There you found a world unto itself, a world to experience and to master. The good news is that you can feel hopeful, even ennobled, by the marvelous care the modern hospital can offer through devoted, hardworking staff more likely than they were in the past to look at you as a whole person rather than a lung or breast or set of bones.

The bad news is that, as in many large organizations, things do not always proceed precisely as planned; you can be confused, even overwhelmed, by the hospital culture—even if you are exposed to it for only a short time. You may feel dehumanized by the scene, no matter how good the institution and how hard its staff tries to care for you, and abandoned when you are told you must leave when you do not yet feel up to it.

Years ago—unless you came in through the emergency room—you were admitted a day or even two days before surgery. Before you reached your room, you went through a battery of tests: chest X ray, electrocardiogram (ECG), blood and urine tests. At times, you were passed from hand to hand efficiently and cheerfully and made to feel like a person, instead of a stiff body, by helpful staff aided by cordial volunteers. Or you could be worried by a disorganized bunch of paraprofessionals of varying quality. On admittance for my first mastectomy at George

Washington University Hospital, one young technician apologized for jabbing my veins repeatedly but fruitlessly after his lunchtime martini (no joke; he had really had one).

Then, I smiled weakly and tolerated such behavior. What was there to do but grin and bear it? But experience has taught me there is indeed something I can do—nothing earthshaking, perhaps, but enough to help me, and the patient who comes after me, and the hospital itself. In brief, I can stand up for myself, acting more assertively and responsibly.

This means I can say to such a young man, not rudely and not aggressively but dispassionately and with respect for him and for myself, "I understand you're not feeling too great. How about finding a colleague to draw my blood?" Or, "I really would feel more comfortable, and you might too, since you're having trouble with my beat-up veins, if you found someone else to draw my blood."

Today you go through the same battery of tests well before admission. For my recent hernia repair, for example, I gathered up my own test results days before my in-and-out surgery—ECG and other information from my internist's office, chest X ray from the radiologist. At the Lombardi Cancer Center, where my oncologist Philip Cohen moved a few years ago, I had some special blood work done.

There, I almost enjoyed having my blood drawn by Colliston Rose, a quiet, precise technician of great competence, who worked in front of a colorful poster of towering craggy mountains captioned "ATTITUDE—A Positive Attitude Overcomes Even the Tallest Obstacles." My blood must be drawn every three weeks these days, and until he was unexplainedly transferred some months later, he always seemed polite and never missed finding exactly the spot to prick painlessly on my dried-from-chemo veins. When I went to the hospital itself for a special test, another phlebotomist greatly impressed me, so carefully did he time the pace at which my blood exited my pricked vein, and so skillfully did he handle my worries.

"Do you think your mind—the way you think—can control how many platelets you make?" I asked him, worried about the "myeloproliferative disease" I now must deal with, probably a

long-term result of the aggressive treatment that saved my life
so long ago. This means my body makes far too many platelets if
I don't take my controlling medication, and since the danger is
thrombosis or stroke, I take it carefully.

He answered simply: "No." But he added: "I'm a Buddhist.
And I think your aura affects what happens to you. And you have
a certain aura." If he had not been so formidable a man, I would
have hugged him.

Of course, you can find other talented people among those working in hospitals today, no matter how varied their resources, and
they can help you feel better about whatever situation you are
in. But you can be puzzled and at times upset simply by the way
the system in which they work operates and by the disconnect
between rosy pamphlets about hospital "caring and curing" and
the realities of what you are experiencing.

Writing on his hospitalization some years ago in his well-
known book *Anatomy of an Illness*, the late Norman Cousins
reported, "I had a fast growing conviction that a hospital is no
place for the seriously ill." The sort of thing he referred to, fortunately, is less in evidence than it used to be: the cool, sometimes seemingly mindless hospital routine: waking you from a
comfortable doze at 9:00 P.M., for instance, to take a sleeping
pill. (When he was a resident, a doctor I know went downstairs
in a crowded hospital to take a much-needed nap on the only
available bed. Finding him there, an officious nurse insisted on
waking him and taking his temperature despite his protesta-
tions: "I'm a doctor—not a patient!")

For Cousins, laughter was the chief answer, not only to the
idiosyncrasies of the hospital routine but to sickness itself. It is
surely true that it helps to maintain your sense of humor, to gen-
tly kid your caretakers as well as yourself. This does not mean
you do not take your situation seriously, just that you don't take
yourself too seriously. It helps to try to put yourself in the place
of the bored staffer who runs her mop bumpily under your bed
while she keeps her eye on your roommate's television "story,"
or the aide, weary from emptying bedpans and other such
chores, who forgets to fill your water pitcher.

With humor and empathy, you'll find it easier to speak up for yourself, tactfully "stroking" the other person before you state your suggestion: "That TV story is absorbing, I know, and a good diversion in the middle of a hectic day. But I'm feeling tired this morning, and I'd appreciate your turning it down while you clean the room." Or, "I know how busy you are doing a hard job, but I need some fresh water so I can take my medicines; I'd appreciate your getting it for me."

Some people fare well with hospital underlings but become tongue-tied when it comes to the higher-ups; sometimes it's the other way around. When your comfort, indeed your life, is in the hands of nurses and doctors, you are often afraid to assert yourself. You fear being thought pushy or uncooperative. You feel the professionals may think you are ignorant or foolish, particularly if you "interfere" with their work or "take up their valuable time" suggesting changes or asking questions.

But this is just the time you should speak up for yourself, asking the questions that are bothering you and suggesting what seems sensible, sticking up for yourself—in the hospital and out of it. In Washington, in pre-dehospitalization days, I was lying in my bed, a chronic patient minding my own business. A nurse came into check on me. "What's the matter with you?" she wanted to know.

I told her I had had an episode of "true vertigo," though she could have seen it from my chart. But my basic ailment was metastatic breast cancer.

"Why?" she persisted. She asked if I had been to the doctor for checkups before I fell ill. I replied in a strained voice that I had been checked every three months over a decade's time but had gotten cancer anyway, in the same breast and the same year of my life as my grandmother. And I had stopped smoking (long ago), did exercises, ate healthy.

Nothing stopped her. My disease seemed to her my fault. She made no move toward me, even to inquire if I needed anything, and observed I should have talked to the doctor about avoiding spread.

My head began to ache, my patience to run out. Perhaps I should have been more understanding about her youth and the probability that she had never seen a long-term survivor—one treated before the options for preventive adjuvant therapies were available. But I simply advised her that indeed I had consulted a good many specialists about avoiding spread and I would rather not discuss the matter any further.

A psychologist/survivor friend of my mom's told me she had taken a leaf out of my book and managed better. When her oncologist repeatedly had no time to answer her questions either at hospital bedside or later, in his office, she asked him to sit down for a minute and said: "I know how important you are and how many people are making demands on your time. But I've got to tell you that the most important thing you are going to do today is to answer my questions."

Shocked, he sat with her for fifteen minutes, allaying her fears. Unaware of the effect of his "busyness" on his patients, he had learned a lesson. And so had she.

Speaking up for yourself can be difficult when you find it difficult to speak at all. When my longtime college friend Betty Randall sensed my apprehension about my approaching tongue surgery, she offered to come up to New York to help out if my husband could not. I thanked her profusely but demurred. It was a minor operation, I told this generous anthropologist/educator who actually enjoys caring for other people; the floor nurses could do the job.

But she insisted, and how glad I was! Though the nurses on the specialized Head and Neck floor answered quickly and usually arrived within relatively short order, I still felt post-op groggy and had trouble finding the intercom and speaking into it through my injured mouth. The nursing office suggested I hire a "companion" (really an aide) instead of a private duty nurse to expedite matters, but I said that would not be necessary because I had a friend who could speak and do for me when I could not—the sort of sleep-in advocate every survivor needs at times! So they wheeled a big reclining chair (instead of the cot we had asked for) into my single room, and Betty, a doctor's widow, stayed the night, fetching the nurse when I needed pain medication, emptying bedpans, cheering me on, and generally turning what might have been an unendurable night into one that was, if not exactly fun, at least companionable.

Sometimes we survivors have trouble fitting into smoothly functioning hospital systems; sometimes we find faulty systems, or even no systems to fit into. Nursing care systems are an outstanding case in point.

Good, continuous nursing care can certainly make all the difference, both in the hospital and outside it. In the early 1980s, when I wrote about "primary care" nursing—in which nurses were assigned a few (perhaps four to six) patients to care for as "total" people from the time they enter the hospital through discharge (and often by telephone afterward)—that patient-oriented system seemed the wave of the future. Instead, it may become an artifact of the past even in pioneering hospitals like Boston's Beth Israel—in danger of becoming a "dead duck," in the words of Pamela J. Haylock (known to everyone as P. J.), immediate past president of the twenty-seven-thousand-member Oncology Nursing Society.

With it may die survivors' dreams of a sure road toward a system in which we have hospital nurses of "our own," who know us as individuals rather than warm bodies in hard beds or cold waiting room chairs. Rather, according to P. J., "there are fewer people who are expected to do more and different kinds of things than we are traditionally educated to do." Albeit necessary, cost-cutting change has brought corporate takeovers, shorter hospital stays, and staffing cutbacks and reshufflings. As a result, says P. J., most RNs (registered nurses) simply do not have the time to do what they want to do: helping survivors from the beginning of their journeys—guiding them as they weigh risks and benefits of various treatments, then on through treatment, helping with new successful medications designed for symptom management related to chemo, radiation, and biologics. And when that treatment ends or is maintained over the long haul, assuring that survivors do not "fall through the cracks" by watching, alongside physicians, for recurrences and monitoring any problems that come up during follow-up appointments.

California oncology nurse Debra Thaler-DeMers adds, "It's an economic thing." Admitting that she is so tired she feels "like a wet noodle" when she goes home after a night shift in which she may have had as many as twelve admissions, Debra, a friend and fellow survivor (Hodgkin's disease) who works out there on the front line on the medical oncology floor at the Good Samaritan Regional Cancer Center in San Jose, is concerned that in this era of managed care, when people are being sent home sicker and quicker and asked to do "more than they are equipped to do" (like changing dressings, emptying drains, and measuring the output), her caregiving capability has suffered.

An RN who earned her B.A. in mathematics, Debra is a licensed public health nurse, which means she can bridge at least one inpatient-outpatient gap by going into survivors' homes and giving chemotherapy. But in the hospital, she worries about the quality of the "team" work she performs helped by often well-meaning but unevenly trained licensed vocational nurses and aides ("cheaper, in the short run" than hiring another registered nurse). For one thing, they cannot give or monitor intravenous medications. For another, the patient may end up on the short end of the stick when such aides fail to report immediately when his or her blood pressure dives to "thirty over nothing" or when the bedpans they empty contain dark urine revealing dehydration.

Nellie Novielli, of the Lombardi Cancer Center, is philosophic. "I think that sometimes you have to see negative changes before things improve," says this RN with a master's degree in nursing. In five years or so, she hopes we will be able to "balance good care with getting the finances back from the insurance companies in order to give good care." But five years is a long time in a survivor's life span.

When I arrived at the Lombardi Cancer Center and they first asked me if I wanted valet parking and then said—going from the ridiculous to the sublime—that a nursing "case manager" would help look after me, I thought that I had died and gone to heaven. I was certainly not disappointed when energetic, knowledgeable, humane Nellie, who calls her role "care" rather than "case" manager, was assigned to me. But as in many other hospital and big institution settings, this idea worked better in theory than in practice. With between six and eight case managers taking care of as many as five hundred patients a week, the sickest survivors take priority; I hardly ever saw Nellie after our initial visit and had trouble getting past her voice mail when I had questions. It could have been worse; in many other hospitals, such "case managers" are relegated chiefly to administrative chores.

Before I knew it, overloaded (and popular) Nellie had been switched off my case to care for other doctors' patients, and I did not see her again until I participated as a mentor in a creative patient–medical student teaching program she and psychologist Julia Rowland had pioneered. Interviewing her later, I found that I had ironically once again been the victim of my own "success" as a long-term survivor who could, the nurses felt, be my own advocate with multiple caretakers (would that it were always so!). "Things move so quickly here sometimes," Nellie explained, "that we don't get a chance to catch up with how quickly patients are moving through the system—and you're considered essentially healthy for a patient coming through."

Good news, in a way. And I empathized with the nurse and her patients, particularly as she told me of the time "when the crunch first started," when a woman on the unit asked for a back rub and no one had time to give her one: "It was so sad—so exasperating, that we laughed about it."

Pain control is another system in constant need of improvement. Writing in the National Coalition for Cancer Survivorship's (NCCS) *Networker*, my friend Fitzhugh Mullan, the physician who cofounded NCCS, gave a "textbook account" of how he, like many survivors, approached his illness in the 1970s with a "bit of macho determination," which together with his doctors' conservative medication constituted "a recipe for pain."

Trying to act as bravely as possible, he toughed out the "morphine every six hours" prescription until he could stand his chest pains no longer and finally prevailed over nurses who insisted on patience and an annoyed resident who argued that he, as a physician, should appreciate the dangers of habituation.

They increased the amount and frequency of his doses; he got relief—without "addiction."

Fitz urged survivors to say *no* to pain and *yes* to pain management, and that is what we, with the help of many caring and enlightened professionals, have been trying to do. But as one of these professional leaders, Sloan-Kettering's Dr. Kathleen Foley, pointed out in the *Journal of Clinical Oncology* in 1995, one-third of patients who receive active therapy and two-thirds of patients with advanced disease report that they experience pain.

This despite national and international efforts to improve cancer pain treatment, including cancer pain initiatives in forty-seven states, curricula as well as guidelines from the federal government and groups like the American Pain Society, the American Society of Clinical Oncology, and the Oncology Nursing Society, and the development of treatment guidelines by the World Health Organization (WHO). The field testing of WHO guidelines, according to Dr. Foley, in conjunction with clinical experience has shown that cancer pain can be controlled using a simple, inexpensive method described as the three-step analgesic ladder (a combination of nonopioid, opioid, and adjuvant drugs titrated to individual needs).

Why, with so much knowledgeable and aggressive attention to new approaches to pain management, did I have to send my friend Betty to get someone to give me pain medication the night after my tongue surgery? Why did I have to persuade the nurse assigned to me how sorely I ached? Why did I have to argue tiredly: No, Tylenol would not do (I had already tried that); I did not want Tylenol with codeine (codeine makes me sick); and not to worry, I'm not going to turn into an addict (finally, she gave me a shot of morphine, and I am here, drug-free, to tell the tale). Why?

Because, Dr. Foley answers, there is a serious flaw in our health delivery system. "No one has time for the pain," she explains, "to gain knowledge about it, to assess it, to treat it, or to teach its proper management to health care professionals and the public." She suggests heightening "pain visibility" by making it a "fifth vital sign" and recording its intensity on the vital signs sheet as a routine practice. Pain is more likely to be treated, she concludes, if you measure and record it.

Alas, it seems visibility is the modern key to change in other crucial areas as well. I had written about patients' fear of hospital errors. I had pointed out, for instance, that several women have told me how they struggled to stay awake before sinking into anesthesia to make sure the surgeon targeted the right breast, and so forth. But, taking my cues from the medical professions, I always prefaced such statements with qualifiers about such mishaps being "rare" or "rare indeed."

One winter evening changed all that. I sat before the television, dumbfounded, watching the unfolding of what came to be known as the "hospital error story." Betsy Lehman, a thirty-nine-year-old health columnist for the *Boston Globe*, had died. Hospitalized for intensive chemotherapy in preparation for a bone marrow transplant at Boston's renowned Dana-Farber Cancer Institute, this breast cancer survivor—a mother of two—had been given a quadruple chemotherapy overdose; another patient who received a similar overdose had become a cardiac cripple (and died some three years later).

I knew Betsy, a respected colleague and daughter of my friend Mildred Lehman, and we shared a passionate interest in patient-doctor communication. We had discussed the crucial importance of what she called "openness and caring, and *listening* . . . patient to caregiver and caregiver to patient." The news of her death, as I later wrote in the *New York Times*, sent shivers through my withered veins—and those of most of the eight million Americans with cancer—not only because the systems for preventing error had broken down or were nonexistent at a top-notch hospital but because a distraught Betsy warned her caretakers repeatedly that something was terribly amiss.

Grossly swollen, vomiting up, as her husband put it, "the lining of her gut," this much loved woman called her caretakers' attention repeatedly to her misery, as did her Dana-Farber scientist-husband. Despite her status as a sophisticated, well-known health consumer, no one listened to her. My sorrow was not alleviated by the ridiculous (for most) TV advice to prevent similar incidents by checking your own chemotherapy dosages or by

Dana-Farber's initial "mistakes happen" attitude. Obviously more than anguished feelings, shattered morale, or noncompliance with treatment is at stake when communications between caregivers and patient break down.

Time, and a whole horde of expert investigators, brought—if not peace—at least a glimmer of brightness to the events of that December 1994 day (not uncovered for several months). Great change took place, not only at Dana-Farber (which eventually shed its defensive attitude and reshaped the institution and the way its patients get care) but at hospitals throughout the country. A new awareness of the danger of errors spurred changes at other U.S. cancer centers. Some three-quarters of the 150 leading cancer specialists surveyed by Dr. David S. Fischer at the Yale Cancer Center in 1996 reported they had reevaluated their chemotherapy safety procedures.

"Betsy Lehman's misfortune has probably saved a lot of other people," said Yale's Dr. Fischer.

Betsy would have liked that.

Still, she would have been the first to point out that our attitude—the way we survivors respond to the hospital culture—can usually influence the degree of our success in taking advantage of the good the hospital offers. Learning to deal with the not-as-good is important as well. Here is some advice for developing such an attitude and negotiating the system I first developed for the NCCS's *A Cancer Survivor's Almanac:*

> *Be assertive.* If your common sense tells you something is wrong, learn to act, not aggressively or rudely, but assertively. This means that if someone jabs at your veins until your arm is speckled black and blue, ask politely but firmly for an explanation and a remedy. If you cannot speak up for yourself, try to get your spouse, a relative, or a friend to speak up for you.
>
> *Know you cannot perform the impossible.* Be equally assertive in dealing with new and sometimes misguided staff efforts to help you avoid hospital errors. If someone suggests that you should check your own drug dosages or

some other aspect of your care, and you wish to do this and feel well enough to try, fine. If not, and particularly if you are alone with no one to speak up for you, respectfully make clear that you are unable to perform what is really your caretaker's job.

Empathize with others. Make an effort to treat hospital staff (and your fellow patients) as you would like to be treated, with respect for them and for yourself. Tactfully "stroke" the aide who interrupts you for no good reason when you are trying to read. This means telling her that you know how busy she is, but that you are not feeling too well and would appreciate a little quiet.

Do not take yourself too seriously. Even as you take your situation seriously, try to keep your sense of humor. When you can laugh and joke and sympathize with others, you will find it easier to stand up for yourself.

Stay alert; speak out; ask questions. Many people are fearful of hospital authority. An extreme example: the patient who is handed a pill he or she feels sure is wrong but fears to ask questions lest doctors and nurses consider her uncooperative, pushy, or "dumb." Remember, no question is a stupid question. You and your caregivers will benefit if you tell them what bothers you and what information you need in order to feel more comfortable (and to be a "better" patient).

If you must complain. . . . When you have exhausted your new assertiveness and things still do not seem to be going your way, by all means complain—to your doctor, to the nursing supervisor on your floor, to the chief nurse, or to the hospital administrator. If your hospital has a patient representative, he or she is a good resource. Present the facts calmly and clearly asking for attention to your problem.

Some survivors almost enjoy hospital stays. Free of the cares of job and household, they savor the (usually) few visitors who hear of their illness before they are sent home, the ministrations of the staff, and the companionship of other patients. A few find their stays harassed and stressful and feel getting home will be an improvement, particularly if they have competent, caring family members and/or friends to help until they get on their own two feet.

Hospitals usually help to plan that reentry into the real world of responsibility and self-care. In the discharge planning process, a nurse, social worker, or some other designated professional works with you to make sure you have the appropriate help and in other ways are prepared to convalesce at home. In looking back at my last two hospital discharges, however, it seems to me I could have followed my own advice more effectively and acted more assertively to learn how to care for my mouth and teeth after the tongue surgery or even how to self-medicate effectively after the hernia repair.

When I received a follow-up letter from Georgetown University Hospital asking me to call them with my reactions to my surgery there, I responded with a call complaining about pain control (I had not been sure what pills to take when the Tylenol did not work). The voice on the phone gave me a brush-off with a curt "You have to talk to your surgeon about that."

Another disconnect: Why did they ask for my reaction only to brush off my response? Perhaps I should have tried harder to answer their letter constructively. But one gets tired, even of a good fight that might help other people.

5 ❧ *A New Subculture*
The New Survivors

The Karnofsky Performance Status (KPS) chart hung on the clinic bulletin board as I was finishing chemotherapy in the early 1980s. When I reported on it in the local newspaper, "they" (the survivor designation for the medical establishment) understood its threatening nuances and removed it.

It no longer appears on the lower right-hand corner of the chart on which the doctors mark my progress, or lack of it, from visit to visit. But I am told they still use it, because, as my oncologist Philip Cohen puts it, for something so subjective, "it reflects patients' health status with remarkable consistency." The other day he told me that since I am "defying the odds and living well on minimal treatment," I now measure somewhere around 90 (*Able to carry on normal activity; minor signs or symptoms of disease*). I am not, for sure, 100 (*Normal; no complaints; no evidence of disease*).

Still, sounds good compared with my postmetastatic period in the early eighties when I measured between 80 (*Normal activity with effort; some sign or symptoms of disease*) and 70 on the KPS (*Cares for self; unable to carry on normal activity or do active work*). Then, I could even slip toward 60 (*Requires occasional assistance, but is able to care for most personal needs*). It could have been worse: 50 (*Requires considerable assistance and frequent medical care*) or 40 (*Disabled; requires special care and assistance*).

"Where's zero?" I asked, when I first saw the Karnofsky chart. It was a half joke, for I knew that the KPS ended with 10 (*Mori-*

bund), followed by 0 (*Dead*). I was familiar with the way doctors "stage" cancer patients according to the size of the tumor and the distance it has traveled in the body. If you are in stage one, the tumor is localized (and small) in the organ in which it originated; if you are in stage four, it has spread invasively to other organs and nodes.

That had seemed like medical gobbledygook. But the even more mundane Karnofsky chart had made me realize I had become part of a new cancer subculture, the subculture of the hanging-in patient. I was not moribund. I was not usually in the hospital. I wrote and browsed through art galleries and drove our car to the grocery store. But I was—face it—not quite well. A sword of Damocles hung over my head, and it felt uncomfortable.

"Where have you been?" asked the tailor when I picked up my coat in late November instead of mid-September. "Listen," I told him, "you're lucky I'm here at all." I feared giving up the now idle stair glide that carried me up and down the back stairs when I had trouble getting around. When the printer asked me if I wanted 500 or 1,000 sheets of business stationery, I hesitated. "One thousand is a bargain," he advised, "but a bargain isn't a bargain if you don't use it." Still, I picked 500.

1998. That printer is long gone, as are the internist who first diagnosed my cancer and a host of other good friends who helped me over the rocks in my early survivorship years. Yet last spring, when a new printer asked me this same question—"500 or a bargain 1,000 sheets of stationery?"—I again hesitated; again chose 500.

The stair glide still rests on my back stairs, idle except when grandchildren I once thought I'd never see try to ride it. I stretch my muscles weekly (well, almost) in exercise therapist Asta O'Donnell's least challenging morning classes (and she forgives my frequent lapses). According to the newer, slimmer status chart provided to my doctors by the Eastern Cooperative Oncology Group (ECOG), I rate somewhere nearer 1 (*Restricted in physically strenuous activity but ambulatory and able to carry out work of a light or sedentary nature*) than 0 (*Fully active, able to carry on all pre-disease activity without restriction*).

Beset by this pain or that worry, I remind myself of nurse Nellie
Novielli's happy opinion of my status: "essentially healthy for a
patient coming through the system."

You guessed it. I am not, in ECOG-speak, *completely disabled* (4). But the Damoclean sword still hovers somewhere up
there—far off in good times, nearby in bad. I am still hanging in
there with a bunch of minor (skin cancers) and major conditions—notably a blood condition that carries the risk for stroke,
which I prefer to avoid, thank you very much—probably a "late
effect" of the strenuous radiation and chemotherapy that saved
my life.

But I am far different from the person I was twenty or even
fifteen years ago. I am part of "The New Breed of Survivors," as a
headline over a late 1980s story I published in the *Washington
Post* put it—"Gutsy, Optimistic, Keeping Their Fingers Crossed."
That headline writer was, and still is, on target: the vast majority of our new breed of cancer survivors expect to survive. Knowing, never forgetting, that some 48 percent of our number still do
not make it, we find hope in the medical progress that has
increased our individual chances for long-term survival—from
successful early detection and conventional "cutting, burning,
and poisoning therapies," as well as from such spectacular
advances as bone marrow transplants. And we have taken comfort in better ways of handling old treatments—like the effective
antinausea drugs now given routinely *before* heavy chemotherapy (a practice that has transformed oncology units, as
nursing leader P. J. Haylock puts it, from "places you could recognize from the sound of people retching" to more ordinary
treatment areas).

Of course, there are exceptions: survivors who, for whatever
reason—from the nature of their cancers to a lack of material and
emotional resources—either do not have the chance to fight or
prefer to try not to dwell on it or adopt a dependent stance ("Just
do it, Nellie, just do it," one such survivor told her patiently
explaining nurse). But most of us live in defiance of cancer and in
affirmation of life—many more, some less successfully than I. We
live out in the open; seldom do I hear of survivors in the closet
any more; oddly enough, two of the few I have known work not

as divas but as artists who fear their diagnoses might somehow stigmatize their careers.

Far more than passive "victims" or even patronized cancer "patients," we are no longer considered damaged goods, told we should be grateful just to be alive, consigned to the role of pitiful poster child at the latest charity ball. Indeed, the standard word *patient* hardly describes us; we are *im*patient.

My phone rings constantly with calls from survivors and their families exploring new treatments, shopping for "the best" doctors (and less often, "best" hospitals), investigating new ways. As we become more seasoned, and gain confidence, we participate with increased vigor in our own treatment, working as best we can with our medical teams to achieve not only more years but more quality control over what goes on in those years—pacing ourselves as we work and play.

Not all but most of us are speaking out, some in the public, political arena and others in smaller but nonetheless important worlds—in the complex and often baffling medical community, for example. We have refused to be put in artificial boxes, to have our lives curbed by inaccurate boundaries, to be considered either cured or doomed in two, or five, or ten years. We want to map our own survivorship journeys.

Dr. Fitzhugh Mullan, National Coalition for Cancer Survivorship (NCCS) cofounder and survivor of an unusual chest cancer (seminoma), started it all in the mid-1980s, when he dared suggest, in the august pages of the *New England Journal of Medicine*, that people are not patients one day (on therapy) and survivors (off therapy) the next. Arguing that actuarial and population-based figures give us cancer "survival rates" but do not speak for the individual patient whose experience is special and not determined or described by aggregate data, he borrowed from medical models to say survivors pass through three "Seasons of Survival": *acute, extended,* and *permanent.*

Remembering the often violent vomiting that followed chemotherapy, the feelings of vulnerability and mutilation that followed the loss of precious body parts, the ups and downs on the therapy roller coaster, trading precious time for treatment and risking treatment for precious time, and the discovery—in spades—of my own mortality (not to speak of worries about my appearance wearing wigs and falsies), I could identify with Fitz's notion of an *acute* stage. But I felt confused about his division between *extended* (read *remission*) and *permanent* (read *cure* or, at least, *sustained remission*) and so sent a letter to the *New England Journal of Medicine.*

After my (then) eleven years as a survivor, I wrote,

> I suppose I should be counted among the "permanent" survivors. But I cannot ignore the fact of my metastatic breast cancer. This is true every day: In my medical life, I have learned to live with a variety of unpleasant pains and illnesses (like shingles or pericarditis) and am still on hormone therapy and maintenance chemotherapy (every two months); in my nonmedical life, I have curbed my ambitions and activities to live . . . a life in which, in a strange way, surviving gets harder with the years instead of easier, because more is expected of you than you can usually deliver.

The journal published the letter (in January 1986), and Fitz responded graciously, writing that he hoped his was a beginning stab at a more sophisticated national effort in the area of cancer survival, to help hanging-in patients achieve lives of quality. He hoped, he said, that others would take up where he had left off.

They have. Susan Leigh, my NCCS colleague and survivor of three different cancers, has analyzed our efforts. Susie, an oncology nurse who now travels the country as a "survivorship consultant," points out that the survivor view is less linear than that of the medical team and seems "more existential and qualitative." Whether we view our experience as a reluctant journey, limbo, or (as I have) living well on borrowed time, we feel, she continues, that we are going through a "continual, dynamic and ever-changing process" as we "live with, through, or beyond cancer."

Thus Wendy Harpham, a Texas physician who had to give up her beloved medical practice as she suffered repeated recurrences of non-Hodgkin's lymphoma, looks at healthy survivors as people able to integrate the reality of their illness into their lives to achieve a "new normal"—sometimes changed from what it was before and sometimes not. Always a survivor, sometimes a patient, but never a "victim," Harpham—who has been among the first patients to be repeatedly treated with genetically engineered biological response modifiers—advises others to obtain sound information—including medical, emotional, practical, and social—to act wisely upon it, and to find and nourish hope.

I like that. I wish I had had access to the concept of a "new normal" when I was on maintenance therapy, feeling utterly bone-weary and having to force myself to ask friends and colleagues to please feed the parking meter or get the Cokes, or yearning for the cane I used briefly after radiation to my hip when no one thought to offer me a seat on a crowded bus. I did not have three little children to look after like the redoubtable "Mommy Doctor" Wendy Harpham, but in our "new normal" state we both learned, in her case to start new, and in mine to recycle, part-time writing (and speaking) careers in which we put our thoughts down for others to read and use.

Similarly, John Anduri, an irreverent Colorado educator/minister and twenty-three-year Hodgkin's disease survivor, writes and speaks to survivorship audiences—including the burgeoning group of men who traditionally have not been taught to deal with the vulnerability, fear, and weakness cancer can bring. He views cancer survival as a circular "Sacred Journey"—in which you pass from Revelation (diagnosis) to Rupture (time of treatment) to Reentry (life after treatment) to Regeneration. In this last segment, you do not come full circle but proceed a bit off the beaten path to a different "well world" in which illness and wellness are integrated, much like Wendy Harpham's "new normal."

Arthur Frank, a medical sociologist, reports in his beautiful book *At the Will of the Body*, that he does not want to generalize his experience of illness into a set of stages, for "only by recognizing the differences in our experiences can we begin to care for one another." Still, this Canadian survivor of both testicular

cancer and a heart attack does feel that since he only hit the surface of his heart attack experience (never referred to as "HA"
though cancer is often called "CA"), he really did "bounce
back," while with cancer, he had "to sink all the way through
to discover a life on the other side."

Frank's "life on the other side" sounds like Harpham's "new
normal" or Anduri's "regeneration" to me.

The new population of survivors hanging in there can be found
everywhere, as I wrote when I prepared the Cancer Survivors'
Bill of Rights—in offices and factories, on bicycles and cruise
ships, on tennis courts and beaches, and in bowling alleys. You
see them in all ages, shapes, sizes, and colors, usually unremarkable in their appearance, sometimes remarkable for the way they
learn to live with disabilities.

Newspapers, magazines, and airwaves seem full of stories of
gallant young survivors. Vacationing in Delaware, I read in the
Wilmington News Journal about Terrie Chrzanowski, a twenty-
year-old who wrote regular dispatches to the paper during her
three and a half years as what she called a "cancer warrior."
Unlike some people, Terry said, cancer never changed her; it just
"more firmly intensified me." Again, my daughter-in-law sends
me a clipping from the *Boston Globe* by another young journalist, Karen Avenoso, who goes ahead with her wedding cere-
monies despite harsh treatment for Ewing's sarcoma—dancing,
eating, and posing for every photo, praising her husband ("other
men I have dated, even loved, would have fled the country").

Such valiant young people pull our heartstrings; no wonder
American Cancer Society media relations director Joann Schel-
lenbach reports that press—particularly television—people seek
them out to illustrate different stories with compelling, often
tragic examples. A bit exploitative, in a way. For the surprising
truth (of which the public is largely unaware) is that the vast
majority of cancer survivors are older people. Testifying before
the President's Cancer Panel (PCP) in 1997, experts pointed out
that more than 60 percent of all cancers occur in the sixty-five
and older age group, and many cancers (lung, rectum, stomach,
bladder, pancreas, colon, prostate) occur even more frequently.

An unfortunate part of this "aged sixty-five plus" survivorship picture: historically, there has been a consistent age-related bias in the care of these older men and women, who often are reluctant to speak up for themselves or even have their children and grandchildren speak up for them; as a result they have been less likely to be diagnosed early and treated appropriately. Surgeons, for example, have preferred to offer breast-conserving surgery, with its potential for improving body image and quality of life, to younger rather than older women with breast cancer; they also have failed to include radiation therapy as part of the treatment given to older women (true across the board, without geographic variation). And one mid-1990s study showed that women sixty-five and older are less able than other women even to *name* a treatment for early-stage breast cancer and also less likely to name lumpectomy as a possible treatment option. (But once properly informed, these women chose lumpectomy with radiation therapy over mastectomy two to one.)

Now, happily, as the nation struggles to make greater progress in the cancer wars, more attention is being paid to this older group, whose numbers, after all, will only increase in the next century. Researchers and administrators are focusing more on their particular problems, including the safety and effectiveness of the drugs they take and the procedures they endure, the multiple tumors and other diseases they suffer, their lack of inclusion in clinical trials, and the amount of untreated pain they bear. Sitting on an advisory committee to a government-funded breast cancer team at the Lombardi Cancer Center studying optional treatments for older women nationwide, I was pleased to note a dramatic change: preliminary, unpublished results seem to show increasing rates of breast-conserving surgery for older women (though there may be other undertreatment issues involved, particularly in those less than eighty years old).

Similarly, those so-called special populations—the diverse racial and ethnic groups whose different cultures (or collective memories) affect the way they handle cancer—have historically suffered special difficulties along their journeys—be it the result of nurture, nature, or community attitudes and circumstances. I first became aware of this at an early NCCS assembly in Los

Angeles, where I heard geriatrician Dr. Al Siu (now at New York's Mount Sinai Medical Center) tell of his problems as a member of an Asian American subculture, in which there is a tradition of family-oriented support that looks for an external cause of cancer in an effort to ward off the taint of disease. Other panel members chimed in—a Hispanic woman spoke of the trouble she had expressing her despair and sorrow to her fearful Hispanic family; an African American survivor from a small town found it difficult to find support, either in her family or community.

Since then I have attended several "multicultural" conferences addressing the needs of groups for whom the distinguished chairman of the PCP, Harlem Hospital Center's Dr. Harold Freeman, has urged more research "in order to give future populations the hope of conquering cancer, even if they fall into a group for whom there are currently few answers." Like Dr. Freeman, you cannot be complacent when you hear how unevenly different cancers affect different groups—San Francisco Bay area data presented to the panel, for instance, showed stomach cancer incidence very high among Koreans and Japanese (though low among Filipinos) and the highest lung cancer rates among African Americans (but increasing in females of all ethnic groups).

And I have been intrigued by various traditional cultural views of health—the Hispanic *fatalismo,* for example, which results in fewer efforts at prevention and attempts to seek care. Or the belief in several cultures—which may change as younger generations replace their elders—that suffering is a test of personal strength; hence treatment may be sought only when a condition interferes with daily obligations (see chapter 8).

It blows my mind when I consider the stamina and guts of most new survivors I have known, whatever their age and cultural background—at every season of their journey, on or off center stage. As a passionate sightseer, I often meet them traveling, be it in Shanghai or Seattle. On a recent bus trip through Great Britain far up in the Scottish Highlands, a woman from Chicago and another from Queensland, Australia—both breast cancer survivors—leaned across a hotel table to clasp hands, sisters found abroad. And a cool, mustached New Englander admitted —a bit shyly but firmly—that he, too, hangs in there with us after a bout with colon cancer.

Back home, I find an e-mail note from Brad Zebrack, a thirteen-year Hodgkin's disease survivor now studying for a Ph.D. in social work and sociology in Ann Arbor. It's a decade since Brad and his wife, Joanne, pedaled eleven thousand miles from San Francisco to Boston and Miami and back to encourage fellow survivors and show that there can be a life after cancer—and that it can be exciting and fun. Midway on their rigorous twenty-eight-state Bike America schedule, Brad reported that riding up steep hills and mountain passes reminded him of his chemotherapy motto: take one day at a time. Even today he reports that parents of young adults and smaller children who've had cancer say they want their sons and daughters to meet him because seeing him healthy and living a quality of life gives them hope.

Similarly, other survivors bicycle or trek across this and other countries to dispel the notion that cancer is an enduring problem: asked how it feels to have leukemia as he started out, Sloan-Kettering patient and volunteer Bob Fisher once answered, "I'd rather have a Danish!" But he couldn't say he felt anything but fine. Lymphoma survivors especially seem to turn up as hardy bicyclists and Outward Bound participants; they tend to feel well when they are in "remission" (a necessary medical word I dislike, because it implies probable recurrence) in contrast to the breast or bone cancer survivors who can be racked with arthritic aches and pains.

As I write, no first or second ladies like Betty Ford, Nancy Reagan, and Happy Rockefeller, no Supreme Court justices like Sandra Day O'Connor or presidential candidates like Bob Dole or Paul Tsongas star in the cancer news. But Orioles outfielder Eric Davis is up at bat, and his cancer is out there with him, though the doctors removed the tumor and treated him with chemotherapy. "I love to play the game," the baseball star confesses." I'll play hard and what happens, happens."

A philosophical acceptance, a feisty fighting stance, and a sense of humor all help. In a doctor's office, I come across a compelling piece in *Glamour,* wherein Wenda Wardell Morrone tells

how her eight-year bout with ovarian cancer had helped her set
goals, dye her growing-in-again hair red, write murder myster-
ies, and marvel at bushes, trees, and, each spring, daffodils.

A fighting Senator Hubert Humphrey, for whom my husband
and I worked at different times, pointed out that if you start taking not your disease but yourself too seriously, you lose perspective. On a holiday in the Caribbean, he told friends, "What a
wonderful place this is! They've got Greta Garbo who doesn't
talk to anybody and Hubert Humphrey who'll talk to every-
body."

Many of us have trouble laughing at ourselves when fate has
dealt us cruel cards. Not Barbara Boggs Sigmund, however, a tall,
blonde, smart, and sassy and unbelievingly courageous poet/
politician who lifted every survivor audience she addressed.
Barbara, once mayor of Princeton, New Jersey, wore flashy eye
patches to cover melanoma's aftermath—white satin or black
checked or dotted pink to match each of her outfits. In November 1989 on a train from Washington, D.C., to Trenton, New Jersey, she complained wryly, in "Ode to my Cancer-Ridden Body":

> Hey, old buddy,
> When did you decide
> That you and I aren't
> Best friends any more?
>
> I had learned
> To
>   strut
>   your
>   stuff
> As well as I could do,
> Though face it, dear old friend,
> You and I weren't getting
> Younger, though I
> Covered up that fact
> As best I could,
> For you, old thing,
> As well as, dear,
> For me.

Don't misunderstand; though upbeat, most new survivors
have been through too much simply to put on a happy face. They
get on with it, according to their beliefs and values, trying in
their different ways to give something back in exchange for
what's left of their new lives. Making research calls for this
book, I became reacquainted with one of them—Liza Fues, a
lawyer and fellow double mastectomy survivor dispensing information on cancer legislation for an applied research and techni-
cal services company serving federal public health agencies.

First diagnosed in 1985, Liza married in 1987, graduated from
law school in 1990, gave birth to a daughter in 1996, and is
expecting a second child. "I enjoy motherhood tremendously,"
she reported, "and find my daughter a constant source of amaze-
ment." But even while she and her husband discuss baby names,
wallpaper a new bedroom for their daughter, and concentrate on
living their lives together, worrisome thoughts intrude periodi-
cally: "How much time will I have with my children? Will I see
them graduate from high school? Have children of their own?
Will I live long enough so that they will remember me?"

Liza "gives something back" to her cancer-related work and to
her family. National Breast Cancer Coalition board member
Christine Brunswick speaks of the "passion and commitment"
her colleagues (often very nervous lobbyists at first) have shown
when demanding, not asking, for increased research funding for
breast cancer and levels of awareness of their disease. I shall
never forget that quintessential survivor Sylvia Cooper, chic,
vibrant despite tough recurrent treatment for ovarian and colon
cancers, answering the phone with a hearty "Praise the Lord!"
instead of the more mundane "Hello." At national meetings, she
infused herself with the nutrients she needed, and she encouraged others, particularly African American women, for whom
she founded Cancer Links All Surviving Sisters (CLASS) in New
Jersey.

As for me, I do the crossword puzzle every morning, to prove
to myself that my brain still works. By being candid and open
about my illness, I, too, try to encourage others to be strong, in
control, independent—and in so doing make my experience useful to others and more acceptable to myself. But like National

Race for the Cure survivors' award winner Ellen Passel, who objects to being regarded as a "candidate for sainthood," I am vaguely embarrassed when people compliment me on being "somehow noble and righteous," or whatever. I know I'm not all that courageous when I stay away from the people who depress me with "downer" remarks ("Natalie! You're still around!") or seek the company of those who seem to accept me, flaws and all.

And I was amazed, absolutely amazed, when Tom Fahey, encapsuling my medical history for another physician a few years ago, said, "I think we can safely say that her breast cancer is no longer a problem." Wow! I'd been his patient for twenty years and never heard him say anything like that before.

Like Liza Fues, worrisome thoughts are not "the focus of my days." Still, also like Liza, I know the other, darker side of the survivorship coin: though old problems may diminish, new ones confront us as we work to create a post-treatment, or, more accurately, post–acute treatment lifestyle that is realistic and comfortable for us. In the past, this has often been hard work because our caretakers, and indeed, the larger society, have not paid much attention to the quality of our lives over the long haul. So we have at times felt like fish pulled out of dangerous waters and left to flounder on slippery piers.

Take fear of recurrence. I used to feel ashamed of myself when I worried about a new ache or pain: Did that hacking cough mean "it" had gone to my lungs? Or did the tingling in my leg mean "it" had blocked my nervous system in some sly way? Is the pain shooting down my arm bone cancer—or a "normal" bursitis treatable with a shot of cortisone? Now I know that such fears are universal: every survivor has to struggle to keep his or her spirits in the face of nagging anxieties. So I try not to deny—but to live with each change calmly a week or two before I bring it to the doctor.

In this I am helped by the attention behavioral scientists have begun to pay to "quality of life" issues. Psychologist Julia Rowland, for example, who has directed the Psycho-Oncology Program at the Lombardi Cancer Center, has identified certain events or conditions that can serve as "trigger points" for fear of recurrence. The sort of "suspicious symptoms" familiar to me, especially those that may mimic symptoms experienced with the original illness (like bone pains), lead the list.

According to Rowland, any change in your health, but particularly weight loss or fatigue, can trigger fear. So can "anniversary events" or dates that mark the course of your illness, such as the time of your original diagnosis or surgery, or scheduled follow-up visits and procedures. Oddly, the end of treatment, which should be a joyful time, can instead trigger anxieties about the loss of a supportive environment or the effectiveness of ongoing monitoring. So, too, can hearing about the death or even recurrences suffered by fellow survivors, be they family members or friends or even high-profile celebrities you have identified with but never met.

And as time passes, and as we live longer and medical science learns more about cancer treatment and its results, "fear of late effects" has begun to haunt us, too. Tough treatments like the "mantle" chest radiation given my colleague Susan Leigh years ago for Hodgkin's disease, or the Adriamycin chemotherapy that so dramatically turned my breast metastasis around, can cause, down the pike, "iatrogenic" (physician-caused) troubles far worse than hair loss or nausea—breast cancer in Susie's case or pericarditis (an inflammation of the lining of the heart), among other conditions I've already belabored, in mine. Not happy trade-offs, but ones we survivors usually feel we absolutely have to risk.

Noting that cancer surgery, radiation therapy, and chemotherapy can all produce late effects—ranging from changes in the blood due to depletion of stem cells to vascular damage in irradiated blood vessels—Dr. Wendy Harpham urges cancer survivors to have routine checkups even when they feel well to discuss lifestyle factors (such as the use of sunscreen lotions) with their doctors. Conscious that up until now such follow-up care has been left in the hands of individual doctors (except for patients in a National Cancer Institute [NCI] clinical trial), survivors are urging a more standardized, organized approach to follow-up care in follow-up clinics for all survivors similar to that used in pediatric survivor care.

The University of Texas M. D. Anderson Cancer Center has created just such a Life After Cancer Care (LACC) clinic in Houston. Headed by internist Rena V. Sellin, LACC was developed to serve former cancer patients considered free of disease and being cared for by primary care physicians, no matter where they received their initial cancer treatment. Staffed by experts on health problems that can occur years after someone has been treated for cancer, it aims not to "take over" patients from community doctors but to work with them as a resource in providing long-term care, through consultations, checkups, medical and psychological counseling.

LACC-like clinics on the lookout for disorders such as osteoporosis and lymphedema in long-term breast cancer survivors, or heart and hormonal problems in childhood cancer survivors, do not yet exist on a nationwide basis. But the fact that medical scientists have begun to turn their attention to the study of survivorship has been a source of great satisfaction to all survivors, particularly, perhaps, to those whose needs have not been adequately addressed in the past.

Many of us joined in a celebration ceremony on the White House lawn a few years ago when President Bill Clinton announced to an audience of survivors, their friends, and supporters that the NCI had established an Office of Cancer Survivorship (OCS), headed—as might have been expected—by an expert in pediatric survivorship, Dr. Anna Meadows.

As the first director of the office, this physician focused her attention on the physical, more than the psychological, problems of survivorship. Yet ten years ago, when I did a story for the first issue of NCCS's *Networker*, the NCI spent less than 1 percent of its budget on what it then called "behavioral research." Now we glory in the fact that under the leadership of newly named OCS director Julia Rowland, the NCI will spend some $15 million over five years (in addition to the $20 million already earmarked) for new research into the physical and emotional well-being of cancer survivors. Dr. Rowland, an engaging redheaded psychologist and longtime friend from the days in which we both served on the NCCS board, emphasizes her interest in studying the role of resilience and optimism—some call it "fighting spirit"—in survival more than identifying the impairment or deficits caused by cancer and its treatment.

So we move forward. As we do so, it is important to remember that no matter how slow the journey, we cannot make it without each other, and without a measure of support from the larger society.

6 ❧ Tools and Crutches

Harry, the blind jogger. I met him where I least expected, in a film shown at a conference held by Washington's St. Francis Center (which deals with the problems of life-challenging illness, loss, and grief). In the film, he ran a race, yoked arm-and-arm to Mike, a fellow runner.

Both were men of indeterminate young age. Both wore conventional jogging outfits. Harry wore a sign saying "Blind Man." Both concentrated intensely on the race. As they threaded their way through a scenic but twisted trail, they discussed the pitfalls confronting them. No rock or boulder or thorny branch escaped their analysis. They planned their strategy ("We're splitting off now").

Dr. Charles A. Garfield led the discussion following the film at this conference addressing the psychology of survival. A clinical professor at the University of California Medical School in San Francisco, he founded and headed the SHANTI project, in which some eight thousand volunteers have served more than two thousand patients a year with life-threatening illness (since 1984 largely HIV-AIDS). "What is real help?" he asked an audience composed largely of counselors and therapists whose daily job is to give it. What energies, what "coping styles" can be used to help a fellow human being, blind or ill?

Harry had electrified the audience. So had his helper, for obviously Harry could not have run the race alone. Even his blunt sign, "Blind Man," was not enough. He needed the eyes his yoked partner shared with him to maneuver the trail. More, he needed the sense of mission they shared—the will to run, to take risks, perhaps even to win the race. He needed to trust his partner, and he needed his partner's trust in his own ability to make it, much more than pity for the fact that, unseeing, he might stumble and fall by the wayside.

Like Harry, every survivor needs help in dealing with the treatment choices and other mighty issues facing him or her, be it at the beginning, middle, or end of the journey. Alone, like that most macho of heroes, prostate cancer survivor General H. Norman Schwarzkopf, we survivors can feel isolated, hungry for information but unable to find it. As California oncologist Dr. Ernest Rosenbaum once put it, we need "tools and crutches"—different according to our diverse needs and values, but tools and crutches all the same. I do not care who you are, or how much money, or status, or inner strength you can muster. You need help.

When I was first sick with cancer, it was not easy to find such help. "Should I go to a psychiatrist?" I asked my surgeon when we discussed my postmastectomy blues. "If you know one you have a relationship with, that would be wonderful," replied Dr. Calvin Klopp, a senior physician in a city with one of the highest ratios of psychotherapists to patients in the country. "But I do not know any I want to recommend. I knew one who was good with cancer patients, but he moved away."

Dr. Klopp is retired now, and in retrospect, his approach seems old-fashioned, but he was a competent, humane specialist in what he called "north of the border" cancer (of the chest, neck, head, and skin). What he was telling me, I think, was that in his broad experience, conventional help tended to force patients to face reality, and reality—at that point—might not be all that therapeutic. But I persisted, explaining that I had called the local American Cancer Society to see if I could get counseling from one of its "Reach for Recovery" volunteers for breast cancer patients, only to be told I needed to be referred by my doctor.

But this doctor again shook his head. "If I could screen all the volunteers, it would be all right. But I cannot, and I've seen too many of them hanging up the crepe."

Surely, this good doctor would not, in fact could not, make such a remark today. For the world has turned over many times in the past quarter century; now, it sometimes seems to me, there has been a support explosion out there, which includes countless veteran survivors helping countless rookies. As the amount that medicine can offer has increased, so has survivors' need for emotional support as they seek information and go through treatment. And it often continues as they find themselves alive—different, perhaps, but alive nonetheless —and having to make undreamed-of choices and set altered goals.

Cancer survivors and their loved ones can choose among a host of supporters. You can find them in a variety of "peer support groups," based in hospitals and medical centers and in organizations out in the community, led by health professionals or by survivors themselves (sometimes by a professional who is also a survivor). And you can find them among many individual counselors, be they social workers, nurses, psychiatrists, psychologists, or trained volunteers who are often survivors with the same kind of cancer as yours.

With optimistic, resourceful, realistic help, you can gather the information you need, analyze it, and come to understand it. In this way, you can get a handle on whatever you fear, keep your balance, and regain your sense of self-worth and self-esteem. Even with such help you may not achieve everlasting equanimity; few people can do that. But you can sort out your options and figure out how you can bring your distress within tolerable limits and spend your time most meaningfully. You can, in short, feel safe—or safer than before.

Of course, not everyone can take advantage of offers of help. Some disdain it altogether and choose to tough it out alone. Others, like a hospital roommate I once had, prefer to rely completely on their physicians. "If I had a problem," she told me, "I'd take it to my doctor. That social worker is too nosy." Very early on, I, too, was wary of support groups, fearing their members might intrude on my privacy or burden me with still heavier problems than my own. I was wary, too, of therapists who might try some weird way of laying hands on me.

But with each passing year, I have grown luckier at getting effective help and more savvy about what I need and when. In the beginning, I consulted a traditional psychiatrist, but one flexible enough to talk as well as listen, even to make suggestions and visit me, both in the hospital and at home (carrying a green spider plant that brightened my stairwell for many years). He helped me particularly with close-to-the-heart problems—my family, who loved me but tried to overprotect me, or my colleagues, who could not quite take my candor about my cancer, or the work I longed to do but could not muster the strength to tackle.

Then, in the middle of a dark hospital night after my cancer had begun to spread widely, a nurse caught me crying in my bed at Sloan-Kettering. She asked what was the matter, and when I grumped, "Nothing," she suggested that I see Sister Rosemary Moynihan, the social worker on the floor. I argued, "I've been through all that. I've seen a shrink. I don't need any Sister Rosemary."

But I hurt, and finally, a bit curiously, I allowed as how I'd like to see the good sister—once. She came in the next morning, and I consulted her for years thereafter whenever I got the chance. At first, I could not look at that angelic face without weeping. She helped me see that I wept because I was for the first time recognizing—mourning, as it were—the progress of my disease. After a while, I was able to discuss calmly with her the radioactive rays chasing the cancer around my body, or the poisons about to be poured into my system. "Adriamycin," she told me, "is called the red devil," and we talked about how that devil might turn into a red angel for me (it did). We talked, too, about what measures I could take if this potent drug nauseated me.

Change, sometimes good, sometimes not so good, has affected this whole scenario. Today, medical progress in the shape of the routinely prescribed drug ondansetron (Zofran) would preclude much prechemotherapy counseling about the management of nausea (though not of alopecia, or hair loss, or a multitude of emotions, such as anger or dread). But you would probably not be in the hospital long enough to meet a Sister Rosemary—if you were there at all.

Still, you can find diverse health professionals in the community, who can act as a sort of liaison with the strange new hanging-in cancer subculture you now inhabit. They can help you integrate the odd world of platelets and prostheses (or now, reconstruction or implants) into your life and make you feel safer in dealing with it. Some can use their considerable community skills in helping you in a practical way, just as Rosemary helped me find a comfortable temporary apartment near Sloan-Kettering. Here my husband, children, and New York friends could visit me while I completed a short radiation course at the hospital outpatient clinic.

Back home, as I grew a bit more open to the notion of accepting help, I found a support group in which I felt comfortable. Led jointly by a psychiatric nurse and a social worker (two leaders can help each other pick up verbal and nonverbal cues as to what survivors need and want), it met weekly in a windowless room adjacent to the hospital cafeteria for a discussion of mutual concerns. Some problems the leaders helped us air seemed weighty at first: Why take on the loss of a testicular cancer survivor's balls when I had enough handling my lost bosom? But I came to look at the group's concerns differently. The heavier they were, the more ordinary mine seemed. As one elderly gentleman put it, "I felt sorry for myself because I had no shoes until I met a man who had no feet." Eventually I got a real lift when two women who had been through bilateral cancer surgery told me how much more balanced and comfortable I would feel after my second mastectomy.

Catherine Logan-Carrillo, the founder of People Living Through Cancer in Albuquerque, New Mexico, who has facilitated a multitude of support groups, explains that "something very special happens when people facing cancer turn to one another for help." I agree. It is amazing how that gnawing feeling in your stomach goes away when other survivors tell you some of their friends avoid them, too; it's not just miserable old you who feels alone. Or that they, like you, had to tell a mother or an aunt not to call every minute to ask how you are doing.

I have visited Catherine, the National Coalition for Cancer Survivorship's (NCCS) cofounder and first executive director, on her half-acre Albuquerque homesite, where she and her husband, Tino (a prostate cancer survivor), tend a lush flower and vegetable garden and care for her horse, Magic, and a number of cats and dogs. A nineteen-year survivor of invasive cervical and now three-year survivor of metastatic breast cancer, she led People Living Through Cancer into national prominence as an innovative peer support organization that pioneered work with survivorship programs among New Mexico's many diverse populations—particularly Pueblo Indians.

It's hard *not* to talk about peer support with Catherine, who became an authority on the subject before she retired at the end of 1997. She appreciates the many different forms such support can take—groups for survivors and/or family members (organized by age, or kind of cancer, in hospitals or in the community), weekend or week-long retreats, one-on-one consultations, telephone hotlines, newsletters, and computer exchanges, as well as large annual meetings, celebrations (like Survivors' Day), and conferences. But she is a particular advocate of peer support groups in community-based, freestanding organizations like her own, which she feels achieve more powerful results than those organized and led by sometimes overworked and/or under-involved nurses or social workers in busy hospital settings.

Some argue that even when a survivor-led group is well structured and planned, empathetic and well-trained professionals can bring a certain amount (but not too much!) of distance to the job and so waste less time than patients going through an emotion-draining experience. Catherine answers with a quote from an Albuquerque breast cancer survivor, Julie Reichert: "I want to be my own expert." She believes groups are most empowering when they are led by survivors themselves rather than once again turning to professionals for help; peer-led support helps people reclaim a measure of control over their own lives.

My friend Nan Robertson, a dynamic, white-haired journalist who once competed with the best of them as a Pulitzer Prize–winning reporter for the *New York Times*, never knew whether the health professional who led the weekly cancer support group she attended for six months at George Washington University Medical Center was herself a survivor or not. It did not matter; though this social worker barely spoke, you could feel her sympathy and her support—in the group room or when she spoke to you privately about a personal problem.

When Nan, a survivor of horrendous bouts with esophageal cancer and toxic shock, joined this group, she knew she was not a stranger. After all, as a veteran member (and chronicler) of Alcoholics Anonymous, granddaddy of all peer support groups, she was used to the group mode and found it powerful. She knew "you are forgiven in that room; no one judges you." What's more, she found it easy to speak openly and to express her anger and her fear, as well as listen to the feelings of others. From other group members' heroic struggles with life-threatening illness, she regained her own courage and ability to laugh and see the positive side of events—an ability that had waned during a long postoperative depression; she returned to work (as a journalism professor) and to a rich and fast-paced life.

So it's different strokes for different folks. Whether you agree with some professionals' no-nonsense approach that we survivors get the least threatening help from the most authoritative experts able to stress that cancer is a very individual thing (and what happens to one person may not happen to another), or with survivors who feel that facts without face-to-face peer bonding and mentoring can bore and befuddle, finding the right group, one that suits your values, your beliefs, and your physical and financial situation, feels, as Logan-Carrillo puts it, "a little like coming home."

Resources and attitudes differ in different places. I've heard of a California breast cancer support group in which a social worker/survivor leader encouraged participants to disrobe, bare and display their chests, and so decrease their feelings of isolation and unacceptability. Such a practice might appall people in a more staid East Coast city; I cannot imagine its taking place, for instance, in a group such as those conducted by Sloan-Kettering's Post-Treatment Resource Center (where a brain cancer survivor wrote Director Karrie Zampini that without appearing "greedy," he wanted to ask for more cerebral therapeutic work-shops because "you offer lifeboats—I survive to flourish").

Another example: When I called CAnCare in Houston, a Texas city with a population of four million enjoying the services of some seventy cancer support groups—including those run out of the renowned M. D. Anderson Cancer Center—I was welcomed with a soft, southern-accented "Thank you for calling CAnCare. We are a volunteer cancer ministry; we believe everyone who has had cancer needs a friend who has walked in their shoes." This was the voice of Anne Shaw Turnage, longtime survivor of colon cancer (with metastases to the liver), who founded the organization and served a seven-year stint as its first executive director.

In partnership with some thirty-two churches Anne, a professional educator, and her pastor husband, Mac, recruited and thoroughly trained 500 volunteers to work one on one with some two thousand cancer survivors and their families. These volunteers, matched with referrals according to cancer site, age, gender, and family situation, provide long-term support and encouragement based on shared experience. CAnCare feels this type of kind, caring, nonthreatening friendship—in which trained volunteers listen, cry, pray, show affection, and even run needed errands for survivors—creates an atmosphere in which survivors can feel comfortable, release and clarify their feelings, and be sure of continued support and follow-up.

In Denver for a family occasion, I stopped by the cozy brick building with white trim that houses another sort of center for cancer support with the same "hugging" feeling of warmth and friendship. But it is a "wellness community," founded by the late Colorado oncologist Dr. Paul Hamilton, perhaps best known as cofounder of the one-on-one peer counseling support program CanSurmount (now part of the American Cancer Society).

In its new home, QuaLife reaches out across the city, networking with hospitals and oncology practices to increase its scope. It offers survivors music, art, and horticultural therapy as well as therapeutic massage and healing touch; under a grant it plans to expand its modest library. Its programs include support groups, one-on-one visits, and Wellness Weekends during which survivor/staff pairs maneuver an obstacle course in the image of Harry the blind jogger; in this case sometimes one is blind-folded, sometimes the other.

At the other end of the spectrum, a freestanding organization, Cancer Care, seems far away from the world of healing touch or trust walks. Headquartered in a busy New York City office building, with offices in New Jersey, Long Island, and Connec-ticut, a social worker staff of forty-five, and a nine-million-dollar annual budget, it offers many professional services: con-ducting support groups, giving individual counseling, dispens-ing information nationwide through modern technologies like teleconferencing, even providing funds for those cancer has left strapped and in need of money for uncovered expenses like med-icines or transportation.

Executive Director Diane Blum, a formidable professional herself, frankly explains that the crux of Cancer Care's philoso-phy is that of a professional service, aiming to help people with all cancer diagnoses. "You should be able to find a doctor you can trust, but you cannot be your own doctor," Diane holds. "Just as you go to a professional doctor, you don't want to turn to self-help when it comes to your social situation or your feelings when you have questions like 'My father is dying and they told me about a hospice, what does that mean?' or 'How do I tell my children?' or 'How can I fill out these insurance forms?'"

Still, she adds, Cancer Care's mission is a personal one: "We don't just send people a booklet on pancreatic cancer or have them talk to a recording. You talk to a human being when you call here."

A few caveats: it's best to shop carefully for the right support for you. You need to know who is leading a support group, for instance, as well as the extent of his or her training, who is in it, how often it meets, and if it is respectful of your confidentiality and organized around issues that interest you—so far as age and type of cancer are concerned. I have met young people who end up inappropriately in an older group of survivors who could not care less about dating problems, and new survivors terrified by the near-death experiences of such people. Men, naturally, might feel dissatisfied with a group composed primarily of breast cancer survivors, just as the most sympathetic women could feel out of place in a prostate cancer session.

A special caveat about confidentiality, an issue dear to my heart since I served as executive director of a national medical records confidentiality commission in the 1970s but which is only now coming to full national attention. Even as we learn to speak and deal openly with cancer, we survivors are realizing that the increasing complexity of the medical marketplace, our reliance on third-party insurers to pay medical expenses, and the exploding use of computers speeding information about our health along the information highway have forced an erosion in the patient-doctor confidentiality we used to take for granted. So we should be vigilant, sensitive to the fact that the physical and emotional information we share in support groups as well as that disclosed to our doctors is kept appropriately private. (Not always the case: a 1993 study showed that more than half of the group leaders responding to a survey reported experience with group members breaking confidentiality, although 87 percent of them said they had briefed their groups on confidentiality principles.)

Another caveat: some groups exist handsomely on paper but not in practice—and this can be true of even national operations that evolve differently in different parts of the country. When my son Jonathan developed Hodgkin's disease, I tried, with NCCS's Ellen Stovall, who once worked for CanSurmount, to find one of that organization's volunteers—a Hodgkin's survivor of roughly his age and interests to visit and counsel with him, enabling him to feel more comfortable about the treatment that lay ahead. After a few days pumping the phone, being transferred fruitlessly from one person to the next, we gave up. Even Ellen's remarkable skill and charm produced only the offer of a middle-aged lady—a Hodgkin's survivor, true, but not the best one to visit Jonathan.

Truly, it takes strong, dedicated, talented leaders, be they health professionals or survivors themselves, to structure groups competently and hold them together. This is increasingly important nowadays, when most survivors stay in the hospital for such a short period that they don't have time to come to terms with their individual situations before they are sent home to monitor themselves—even on sophisticated chemotherapies (with only telephone help from their doctors' offices). In contrast, as I have pointed out, when I had my surgeries in the seventies and eighties, I stayed in the hospital for a week or ten days—a period long enough to take part in a support group on my breast cancer floor in which we patients had time to air our feelings and learn some practical skills (like arm exercises that enabled us to stretch our muscles and so heal better).

As I became a more and more seasoned survivor, I seemed to find the tools and crutches I needed in still larger groups and networks. First, I cofounded a local network of survivor groups and individuals, the Greater Washington Coalition for Cancer Survivorship (GWCCS), in the capital area in the late 1980s; eventually, the late Diane Sheahan, an ovarian cancer survivor and talented community organizer, took up the GWCCS reins and, working with local hospitals, built a viable organization that still produces an outstanding computerized informational newsletter in which local survivors can find what resources they can tap into, when and where.

Moving on, I gained more tools and crutches from many of my NCCS activities, which made me feel better about my own cancer and gave me the chance to give something back to others. Founding and editing the *Networker*, for example, I used my reporting skills to find out what I wanted to know about survivorship and to present this information for others to read and use. By attending and speaking at conferences and meetings around the country and participating as an active board member at the NCCS's annual assemblies, I have continued to meet and be inspired by marvelous role models and tried to serve as one for rookie survivors. And I have taken advantage of countless learning opportunities—whether they be in workshops on nutrition or sexuality or job discrimination or journal keeping.

I remember feeling thoroughly at home at an NCCS assembly where participants wore buttons saying "Cancer Sucks" or "I've

Been Pushed to the Limit" or even "There Is No Such Thing as False Hope." In the corridors, and over a decaf, I have picked up reliable skinny on a host of matters big and small, from how to find chic, durable hairpieces to the whereabouts of certain "best" cancer genetics specialists or authorities on cancer pain management to the implications of a newly enacted health law for the confidentiality of medical record keeping.

Some innovators have begun to use modern technologies to bring the feeling of support and bonding to an even wider audience. Through "The Group Room," a national radio talk and call-in show, one of my NCCS colleagues, Los Angeles breast cancer survivor Selma Schimmel, translates survivorship issues for an estimated twenty thousand listeners in our country and in Canada. A dynamic impresario, Selma, who for many years has led the young people's support group Vital Options, enlists the help of various professionals—including oncologists and mental health specialists—as well as survivors, as she conducts a show in which survivors can meet, talk, take care of one another, and exchange information. When she explains that on her show there are no visual distractions, all you need "is to have your heart and your ears," her enthusiasm is contagious and her show effective, even if it lacks the intimacy of face-to-face support.

Another example of less participatory (with time only for two or three call-ins) but effective high-tech "grouping": I listened, spellbound, on the telephone, along with some 699 other survivors, as Cancer Care experts laid out the facts about breast cancer that has metastasized to the bones. I found it so easy to follow and compelling that I hooked up to other teleconferences. After such a conference on managing cancer pain, one caller, a midwestern survivor who had been told by local doctors that her relentless bone pain resulted from a form of arthritis, was advised by social worker/leader Carolyn Messner to make a follow-up call to Cancer Care. She did, I later learned, and was steered to a Comprehensive Cancer Center she had not known existed just ten minutes from her home. Here she was diagnosed correctly and began life-saving treatment for bone metastasis.

Of course, not all survivors feel at home in a group, be it small or large. They may be plain shy or, for whatever reason, unable to share private fears or discuss personal problems with their peers. Such men and women benefit more from one-to-one counselors who will listen to their words and observe their body language, creating an atmosphere of acceptance that gives them the freedom to express their innermost anxieties and concerns and often leaving them less tense, more hopeful, and feeling better about themselves.

Groups and individual therapists are not, of course, mutually exclusive. During the course of a full but often difficult life that included a tough bout with cancer, one of my friends has seen three psychiatrists (finding one "a disaster" and the other two helpful) as well as participated fruitfully in support groups. As I've hung in longer and longer, I, too, have been helped by individual therapists as well as groups, including a center—the Medical Illness Counseling Center in nearby suburban Maryland —that offers both.

Dr. Stephen Hersh, who founded this center with fellow psychiatrist Lucy Waletzky and named it euphemistically to attract ill people wary of all things "psychiatric," works with a number of different health professionals, from physical therapists and social workers to psychologists specializing in biofeedback or hypnosis. In his book *Beyond Miracles: Living with Cancer*, he stresses the necessity of checking out the experience and training of those who offer you therapeutic services. Explaining that since such therapists combine their natural talents and training to interpret the special dimensions of patient realities with a highly honed sense of timing as to when to attempt an intervention and how, Dr. Hersh points out that their credentials should assure you of their proper education and supervised clinical training.

I agree. This is not the time to fall into the hands of poorly trained people who could take advantage of your vulnerability. This is particularly true because there is such an assortment of therapists and therapies out there for you to choose from. In a 1997 review, "Literature on Interventions to Address Cancer Patients' Psychosocial Needs," authors Vivian Iacovino, M.D., and Kenneth Reesor, Ph.D., surveyed thirty-three studies of various ways—from cognitive therapy and health education to crisis intervention and relaxation training and combinations thereof—in which therapists step in to help survivors, in groups (eighteen studies) and out of them (fifteen studies). The authors concluded that the psychosocial interventions generally had "a positive impact on patients' adjustment and adaption to cancer" but that no particular psychosocial intervention seemed to be significantly more effective than others.

In any event, survivors need to be scrupulous in checking out *individual* as well as *group* "helping" credentials. And I would add that with the increased use of psychopharmacological medicines—largely mood altering drugs that can help you deal with anxiety and pain—you may find it simpler to consult therapists who, if they are not physicians themselves, at least have immediate access to physicians with the authority to prescribe.

How can different survivors tell if they need special support? And if such support is needed, how can caregivers help connect them with the right sort?

"Really, it is normal to be sad if you have a bad diagnosis," according to Sloan-Kettering's psychiatric chief, Dr. Jimmie Holland. "It is normal to be frightened, afraid and anxious about the future. We expect such emotions; they are par for the course for anyone going through crisis and illness."

Dr. Holland, who after more than two decades of work has become the doyenne of the psycho-oncological community, stresses that for some cancer survivors "their sadness is a little more than that"—their mood is down, they don't see the future as very hopeful, they don't feel as well or function as well. And still others—a much smaller percentage usually with a lot of disability and inability to function in their usual ways—feel significantly depressed: "Like I don't want to live any more. I don't have any pleasure in anything I do; I would just as soon not be alive."

Just as there is a kind of continuum for depression, the psychiatrist explains, there is a continuum for anxiety: "It is normal to be frightened, normal to be fearful, but some people become so frightened and so fearful that they cannot function and can become preoccupied with worrying about what will happen next; such feelings can cause their heart to beat fast or make it difficult to breath and concentrate." Wherever survivors are along this emotional continuum, she believes, it is more useful and less threatening to talk about stress and distress than depression and anxiety disorders, and it behooves professionals to find a simple "emotional thermometer" to measure that stress. Using the power of our experience along this emotional continuum, survivors for some years have urged the health care system not only to provide psychosocial services for people with cancer in an organized way but also to consider such services a necessity, rather than a luxury. And spokespeople like the NCCS's Susan Leigh have pointed out that the plethora of services now in existence vary enormously—in some places and some hospitals, it's catch as catch can, and what exists is usually there only for the newly diagnosed survivor.

"We have no systematic follow-up unless we're in a clinical trial," this oncological nurse and survivor of Hodgkin's, breast, and bladder cancers told the 1996 NCCS Assembly. "That's 3 percent of the population or less. There isn't even an exit interview when you come off care."

Now the medical system is beginning to respond to such complaints and to figure out which survivors need psychosocial interventions, as well as when and how these interventions should be offered. At the Johns Hopkins Oncology Center, Associate Director of Community Research Jim Zabora, a tall, genial, tenacious social worker, has led a multidisciplinary group dedicated to finding the answers to such questions. The result is an innovative, integrated program in which staff does not wait for cancer to trigger a crisis in new, vulnerable patients but steps in to identify and prevent it.

Pointing out that survivors, even people at the same stage of the cancer experience, bring different internal and external resources to treatment (like their level of optimism or family and financial support), Zabora says they look at it very differently. For some, with a high level of resources, the disease can feel like a challenge; for others, with a low level of resources, it may seem so overwhelming that it allows little chance for a hopeful survival. And the stress of these vulnerable patients will remain elevated not only at the time of diagnosis but all through treatment and beyond—unless something is done to address it.

Unless something is done to address it. During your first week of care as a cancer patient at Johns Hopkins, you are asked to fill out a one-page questionnaire as part of the registration process. On this "Brief Symptom Inventory," you rate on a scale of 1 (not at all) to 4 (extremely) your level of distress on fifty-three different items from "Nervousness or shakiness inside" to "Nausea or upset stomach" and "Feelings of guilt."

From the answers, which most (about 80 percent) registrants give willingly, staff can measure the distress you are feeling and so determine the psychosocial service from which you would most benefit: educational/informational seminars and one-on-one patient-to-patient support if your stress measures low or "normal"; group support or short-term counseling if you are moderately distressed; and a "mental health approach" if you are experiencing more severe distress—be it psychotherapy or counseling and, for ominous symptoms (like suicidal urges or severe anxiety), specialized help (probably including medication) from a psychiatrist.

With some eight thousand psychological profiles compiled, the Johns Hopkins program has found about 30 percent of the patients assessed to be either moderately or severely stressed and so more vulnerable. This does not mean that the remaining 70 percent need no psychosocial services; program leaders feel everyone could probably benefit from some service, even if the focus was informational. But distress must be measured and vulnerable patients identified and matched to the appropriate psychosocial services quickly.

East Baltimorean Zabora is refreshingly candid about his program's approach. For one thing, he admits he has had to play the "data game"—though he is not fond of it—to convince his own bosses as well as insurance companies and managed care groups that appropriate psychosocial interventions can not only increase patient quality of life but save health care costs. He explains that patients—wanting their doctors to like them and to focus on their cancers rather than their tears—often conceal emotional reactions and medicalize their complaints, telling oncologists not, for instance, about postmastectomy problems with intimacy but about growing aches and pains and trouble sleeping. Instead of referring such patients for counseling, doctors (operating in a fifteen-minute time frame) respond with medications, scans, and tests. Consequently, the bill could rise considerably higher than the $500 that would have been charged for ten counseling sessions.

Zabora readily admits that his program has not done enough to measure distress among long-term survivors: "Absolutely. We know nothing beyond two or three years." But researchers have found an increase in distress, or at least sadness, after three years in bone marrow transplant survivors: "Your first year is strictly surviving the disease and treatment, your second year is your rehabilitation and recovery. Then, you begin to realize what you have lost along the way. You realize that your career has changed; you realize that you are not going to be able to have children. So there has to be some grieving for those losses."

Absolutely. And unless programs are offered to address such concerns, survivors sometimes turn to other forms of support—on the fringes or completely outside the health care system.

7 ∞ Complementary and Alternative Therapies

Quiet. Very quiet. Eight of us survivors, with eleven staff/care-takers, sequestered at a "Cancer Help Program" week-long retreat, left our shoes at the entryway and went about in socks. We read no newspapers in our Georgian brick manor house on Maryland's Eastern Shore, watched no television, and heard no radio. We ate no meat, drank no coffee and, of course, no alcoholic beverages. Although telephones were available for credit card users, they never rang, and we were asked not to use them except when absolutely necessary.

Sitting cross-legged at our early morning yoga sessions, filling my lungs, even my stomach, with fresh air, relaxing, meditating, stretching and twisting aching parts in ways I would not have thought possible, I asked myself why I had I come here, to this warm and fuzzy land of holism, of mind-body connectedness, so late—twenty-three years late—in my cancer journey. Why had I come when I knew myself to be wary of out-of-the-mainstream approaches to cancer treatment? Why had I come when I was apprehensive that, though I might inspire some fellow participants who had not survived as long as I, I might also depress them with the news that cancer can haunt you for many years even after "remission" is achieved? (How I hate that word, with its ominous implications; I wish the powers-that-be would say "cancer free" instead.)

Free of what our yoga teacher, Shanti, she of the beatific face and rubberlike body, called the everyday grocery-list "chatter of the mind," I remembered a friend saying she had felt a "thin gray line on things—sometimes bored, sometimes smiling less," and I knew a similar gray line had been invading my consciousness. Although, happily, my breast cancer "remission" had remained stable for years, I had had to return to the world of hospitals and clinics. Tri- or biweekly blood drawings and even a light chemotherapy pill had had some unpleasant side effects and gotten me down; growing older, having to slow down and see too many of those I love fade, with all that implied, had not helped.

I wanted to ease the pain in my heart (and, possibly, in my postsurgical mouth) and find a greater measure of calm and peace. I wanted, as my friend with the gray line put it, to find a greater sense of connectedness—to my work, to my family, my friends, and community. I thought I just might succeed at this Smith Farm retreat, fathered, like its California parent, Commonweal, by Michael Lerner, Ph.D., as a sort of Commonweal-East. Though this smart and savvy former MacArthur Prize Fellow is a tenacious advocate of assuring survivors the choice of unconventional as well as conventional cancer treatments, he offers no Lourdes-like cures. In contrast, he now insists that such treatments be called "complementary" rather than "alternative" and that all program applicants make sure that their oncologists know and approve of their attendance. Besides, though I do not always agree with him, I respect his work, which is more than I can say of some other heavies in the field.

So I applied (my oncologist could not have cared less), and I was admitted (only after a last-minute vacancy occurred at Smith Farm). I paid out my fee—$1500 for seven days, which, though expensive, does not cover the cost of this labor-intensive program. I was there, and happy to be so, though the floor on which I lay doing my yoga felt a bit scratchy, and the proliferation of beans made me fart. When, after one of Michael Lerner's evening talks on matters complementary, I confessed to harboring a hefty degree of skepticism, he quoted Santayana: "Skepticism, Natalie, is the chastity of the intellect."

If that is so, I responded, I am more damned chaste than I thought. The curly-headed director is nothing if not patient-oriented. And, in his favor, he has not fallen victim to money madness or haughtiness as have some of his peers, despite Commonweal's featured appearance on the Bill Moyers show.

Later on, I realized that the patchwork of services Smith Farm/Commonweal offered to us participants—six cancer survivors (the others more freshly diagnosed than I) plus one spouse and one significant other—reflected the way the government's Office of Alternative Medicine (now Center for Complementary and Alternative Medicine) has classified today's unconventional treatments to provide a structured way of looking at them. We were exposed to a sampling of each (with the exception of two of the agency's seven categories—*Bioelectromagnetic Applications* and the controversial *Pharmacological and Biological Treatments*).

We overdosed on yoga and meditation (*Alternative Systems of Medical Practice—typically ancient approaches*); these were punctuated by readings from East and West, but particularly from Eastern or Indian cultures: from Shanti, for instance, during yoga:

> Watching the moon
> at dawn,
> solitary, mid-sky,
> I knew myself completely:
> no part left out.
>   —Izumi Shikibu

or from Lenore, during Group, "The Five Remembrances":

1. I am of the nature to grow old. There is no way to escape growing old (ring the bell);
2. I am of the nature to have ill health. There is no way to escape having ill health (bell);
3. I am of the nature to die. There is no way to escape death (bell);
4. All that is dear to me and everyone I love are of the nature to change. There is no way to escape being separated from them (bell);
5. My actions are my only true belongings. I cannot escape the consequences of my actions. My actions are the ground on which I stand (three sounds of the bell).

The pace picked up during the week, so much so that I hardly had the chance to walk out along the woodsy nature trail bordering the bay. Never again, I thought, would we participants receive such intelligent, energetic individualized loving care— whether it was Rachel, the cook's sister/aide, asking me how the fiber-heavy vegetarian diet (*Diet, Nutrition, Lifestyle Changes*) was affecting me (I confessed to no longer being my usual constipated self), or Jnani interrupting her skillful every-other-day massage (*Manual Healing*) to compliment me on my writing or suggest that I ask former publisher and therapist Dick Grossman, who, for twenty years, honchoed a Health in Medicine Project at New York City's Montefiore Medical Center, if he knew of any potion to help my sore tongue. He gave me the little bottle of tea tree oil he carried about; it proved soothing, though not curative (*Herbal Remedies*).

Somewhat hesitantly, I signed up for art and sandbox play therapy; when our teacher, Barbara, asked us to draw the worst possible ogre, I produced a credible, if awkward, beast with a large red tongue and wicked claws; she told us to label it "the Critic"—that pesky creature within us that constantly criticizes what we do and tells us we are not good enough to attempt this or that (*Mind/Body Control—use of the senses to enhance well-being*). My Critic was later tacked onto my kitchen bulletin board, in hopes that Barbara's message would continue to rub off on me as well as on my often critical husband.

Central to our week's experience were our daily two-hour morning group sessions with program co-director Lenore Lefer, a compassionate psychotherapist with unruly graying hair, bare feet sporting painted red toenails (more *Mind/Body Work*). On day one, she told us that when the week was over we would all just love each other, and it was true. Standing in a circle at the end of each session, hugging, we bonded. Gradually, haltingly, we eight women and men (whose identities are masked here), ranging in age and point of origin from California to Kentucky, Colorado to Canada, began to speak our hearts.

We wept for ourselves and for each other, for our lost years and body parts, for the young architect who kept her colon cancer secret, even from her little son, for the baker-turned-government-bureaucrat who lost his eye to melanoma (in the operating room he looked up at a blackboard chart and saw himself scheduled to have the wrong eye taken out), for the elegant lady in her seventies whose breast cancer felt less of a problem than her wish for a fuller life, for the former Wall Street whiz who, when he thinks of dying, thinks first of getting his taxes in order but spends hours preparing nutritive capsules for his wife he—and to a far lesser extent she—hopes will help stave off a recurrent ovarian cancer. I said I hoped someone held stock in the Kleenex company.

Though I often listen to tapes that help me relax and even sleep, I had never considered myself terribly good at meditation—those sessions in which you take deep breaths and imagine yourself in golden fields or by peaceful ponds where you can picture your good immune cells eating up the bad cancer invaders. But as we were led by Lenore, the seeming foolishness of this process fell away, and I found my "wise person" in a childhood mansion near a field of flowers. She appeared as my long-dead grandmother at the top of a majestic staircase, wearing her usual lavender dress, ready to help and care for me. The architect's wise person surprised her as *Star Wars'* Yoda, a funny little fellow dressed in yellow who advised her to take one day at a time; for the significant-other lawyer, the wise one appeared as an irreligious Virgin Mary in purple leggings and Birkenstock sandals.

Healing. Healing is what the program is about, not curing (though curing would be nice)—a hard concept for some of us to grasp. Healing, Michael Lerner explained in one of his evening talks on Complementary Therapy, takes place in both living and dying. In the healing process, you go down deep within yourself to find your own special way of responding to your disease and the stress it brings. As you relax in the kind of safe space the program gives you, you may reevaluate your ways and connect with a new wholeness.

Does this sort of healing shift the course of a disease? Michael said we do not know yet, but many feel it can shift the more general nature of your condition, making you stronger at your spiritual core and so encouraged and strengthened.

Well . . . At one of the closing sessions, we were asked to write around six lines of verse starting each one with the same noun, any noun at all. I picked "Healing," and I wrote, a bit irreverently:

> Healing is peeling layers away
> Healing is kneeling day after day
> Healing is funny
> Healing costs money
> Healing becomes thee
> Healing, let's hope, gets to me.

As I drove home from the retreat, the world seemed a honking, hustling, bustling place. Still aglow and relaxed, I lost my way on the back roads of the Eastern Shore but focused in time to hit Route 50 just at the point where a familiar outlet shopping behemoth sprawled at Queenstown. I had my first Diet Coke in a week in a favorite New York deli; it tasted good after all that herbal tea. And in the Liz Claiborne emporium I found a red silk pantsuit with a chic pink collar, ideal to wear with a black turtleneck to my upcoming birthday party. Was it a power suit?

I knew the retreat had been, to use an enigmatic word, a "powerful" experience. I did not think it had changed me in any radical way. But it had not hurt me; indeed, perhaps all that warm love and support and relaxation had helped gear me up for my next writing project (this book). And I felt good.

One of the most challenging, worrisome, and persistent questions in a cancer survivor's life is whether to use unconventional (or unproven or nontraditional) treatments, and if so, how to use them. Call them what you will—and however they are proposed, either in place of your conventional care or in addition to it—you are bound to hear of them and, probably, to be tempted to try them, according to your nature and, I imagine, nurture.

Sitting in the clinic waiting room, talking to the retired nurse down the block, on the phone with a well-wisher or a gravely ill acquaintance desperate for help, reading newspapers and magazines or watching television accounts of holistic or mind-body "cures," one senses there must be something out there in addi-

tion to standard medical treatment, something that might at
least ease your pain and at most help beat back your cancer.

That "something" can appeal to you in many ways and for
many reasons. Looking around, you see a do-it-yourself society,
with almost everyone out there dutifully jogging, working out,
or at least eating "thin" to keep in shape. Curious, you may wonder if a similar self-help approach might make you feel more
comfortable, leave you in better control of your well-being, and
generally improve the quality of your life with cancer. Or you
may have had your fill of the often impersonal nature of modern
high-tech treatment—the technicians who coolly leave you without a word of encouragement, alone in the drafty radiation room,
just another inert body dealing with a mighty machine; the
oncologists without time to answer your questions or who even
fail to recognize you in the clinic elevator; the cancer center that
dismisses you, as one did my beloved sister Ellen, gravely ill
with pancreatic cancer, with a resigned "there's nothing more
we can do for you." (Desperate to live, with little time to waste,
this Ph.D. historian turned to an unknown, if well-meaning,
researcher who promised her an immunological "curative" vaccine produced from her tumor in a basement laboratory in
Yonkers; she died a quicker and probably more painful death as a
result.)

Again, exhausted by repeated "cutting, burning, and poisoning" therapies and fearful of experimental treatments like bone
marrow transplants, you may look wistfully, even respectfully,
at modern versions of mystic and ancient approaches used for
thousands of years by millions of people, such as "traditional"
Chinese medicine or the Indian Ayurveda, with their talk of life
force and spiritual harmony between body, mind, and the environment. You may throw up your hands and ask: "Why not try
something more natural, something that won't destroy my
body's own defenses, something gentle, easy, and hopeful I can
do for myself—like meditating, breathing deeply, and imagining
my good cells conquering the unruly cancer cells, or eating
restorative grains, or purifying and cleansing my system with a
coffee enema?"

Why not?

In the early 1980s, I had discarded my clumsy back brace, which made me sweat and made my clothes balloon. But metastatic cancer had eaten into my upper spine, I had a permanent slipped disk, so to speak, and nagging back pain still kept me constant company. Doctors and the Sloan-Kettering pain clinic had only given me more pills. Small doses of Elavil made my hands tremble.

I wanted competent, not shaky, hands. Seeking new approaches, I consulted a psychologist who specialized in hypnosis and pain control (who had helped a friend give up smoking and others overeating). I had read about hypnosis; I knew a hypnotic state to be an altered state of mind or consciousness. In such a state, I could suspend some of the functions of my conscious, wakeful mind and focus my attention on a few inner realities. I could become more receptive than usual to suggestions or direction.

Could the psychologist help dull my pain? Would I lose control over my mind? Apprehensive, I sat in his office armchair, listening to his soft voice, "Natalie, find a comfortable position. Find something to focus your attention on. I'm going to count from one to three. At one, I want you to do one thing, at two, two things, at three, three things. . . ."

This was not so bad after all. "First take a deep breath and hold it. Breathe in relaxation, breathe out tension." The hypnotic tapes he gave me to practice with at home did not wipe away my pain. Using one, called "glove anesthesia," I could put my hand to sleep by thinking about the last time the dentist gave me Novocaine. But I could not, even in a trancelike state, transfer the numbness to my aching back. Nor could I, using another tape, forget that back by returning to the past and focusing my full attention on a press club trip I had taken to Russia some years before.

Still, the experience did help me relax my tense muscles, and in so doing, it led me further into the land of Holism, whose wild mix of wares had always seemed to me for the birds, or at least for the young, prevention-minded, veggie-consuming counterculturist, not for a middle-aged cancer survivor whose grandmother had gotten cancer at just about the same age and in the same pattern. Here I found herbal teas sitting on coffee tables, acupuncture charts adorning walls. Mellifluous voices on tapes . . . tapes . . . and more tapes . . . an upbeat atmosphere of touching, and yes, even of love.

First names . . . there are few last names in the land of Holism, which originated in the ancient East, renewed under the tolerant skies of sunny California, and exploded in my own darker, more skeptical Northeast, with more of a philosophical than a scientific message: not only can psyche affect soma and vice versa (in malignant tumors and heart disease as well as headaches and ulcers), but we human beings are psychobiological unities, integrated within ourselves and our environments; illness is an alien invasion of the positive harmony between mind and body; treatment is an effort to restore this harmony. Since mind and body work as one, there can be both an internal cause and cure, if only you take responsibility for finding them.

Tentatively, I began to explore that option. In my old khaki pants, I lay on the carpet in an empty living room in a big house off Sixteenth Street, pushing various limbs against the floor and trying to learn from two young teachers of the Feldenkrais method how to increase my ability to use my whole body comfortably. They promised, not a cure, but a new ability to use your entire muscular apparatus, and as a result, more awareness of your movements and so lighter and freer patterns of movement.

I was willing to try moving with more grace and balance and so—perhaps—to improve my health and well-being ("When a person is healthy, it turns out he is not ill," according to guru Feldenkrais). But my teachers lost me completely during an interview in their kitchen after class when, over herbal tea, they scoffed at scientific studies done by "$40,000-a-year researchers." They could not manage, they said, as I squirmed uncomfortably, in the "entrenched experimental paradigm" but preferred one based on "subjective experience." It was not the last time I would hear this sort of suspicious, to my mind unconstructive, chatter in holistic territory.

I tried again. In a Guided Imagery Workshop at the Washington School of Psychiatry, I strained to follow a white-haired UCLA faculty member when she suggested we form different

pictures in our minds and interpret what we saw, like psycho-
analytic patients analyzing dreams. In a simple Bethesda church
I listened as a former atomic scientist talked about "effective
prayer." I gathered that this involved healing yourself by finding
the "LIGHT" and healing others by visualizing the "LIGHT"
in a neighbor. Not for me was the flowery language and rapt
approach ("I release all of my past, negatives, fears, inner self,
future, and death in the LIGHT. . . . I am a LIGHT being").

And at a conference of the same respected organization where
I had met Harry, the blind jogger, I found I could not accept all of
well-known psychologist Lawrence LeShan's profile of a typical
cancer patient: someone who lacked closeness to both parents.
Someone who has suffered a loss. Someone who feels hopeless,
helpless, caught in the web of life who says: "If the egg drops on
the rock—poor egg. If the rock drops on the egg—poor egg." *She is
the egg.* That description—in toto—simply did not fit me, or many
other survivors I knew.

At still another conference held at a local university, the message seemed similar but the scene different. I had come, not to
an ordinary day of lectures and workshops, but to a happening,
featuring two stars, Dr. Carl (a former radiation oncologist) and
Stephanie (a psychologist) Simonton. Before a rapt, adoring,
seemingly uncritical audience of some five hundred people, they
explained how the imagery techniques they had pioneered—
relaxing and visualizing the good cells destroying the bad—could
help us patients participate in our treatment and battle cancer.

The couple (since split) echoed LeShan: rather than striking
out of the blue, cancer develops out of a complex interaction
between personality traits and stressful life events. It particularly afflicts "cancer-prone personalities"—people with poor self-
images and bottled-up resentments, who have trouble forgiving
and forming long-term relationships and, importantly, have lost
a serious love object or life role only months before a diagnosis.
When such helpless, hopeless folks are stressed by a demanding
boss or nagging spouse or whatever, their despair, in a sense, is
turned inward, and the central nervous system can suppress the
immune system, nature's first line of defense against cancer
cells.

Talk of "being gentle with yourself," loving concern, and learning to use tools like exercise, diet, counseling, and playing "smart" instead of "dumb" abounded. But when, at the end of the day, Stephanie stated, before this room packed with cancer survivors, counselors, and other supporters—many of whom had been to hell and back—that she hoped a cure for cancer would *not* be found, as a cure for polio had been, I was shocked, and so was a friend, a fellow survivor. But unbelievingly, most of the audience seemed to accept and admire the speaker's cruel reasoning that such a vaccine-like cure for our sufferings would mask the societal issues involved, such as the stressful ways we bring up children or the manner in which we allocate medical funds. One woman responded, "Thank you, Stephanie, for your excellent presentation and your guts."

When he arrived at the Simonton Center in Temescal Canyon north of Los Angeles some years later, actor/leukemia survivor Evan Handler has reported in his compelling book *Time On Fire*, he felt as though he had escaped one lunatic asylum (the hospital) only to enroll himself in another. But, like me, he developed confused and mixed feelings about the New Age goings-on, admiring Carl Simonton and his message and methods for increasing control over one's own life (and disease) but objecting to the way he and his peers promoted their philosophies as pat formulas or equations. In the end, the young actor—worried about the possible results (blistered flesh, bandages and ointments)—refused to join in the seminar's closing fire walk, in which some participants proved their dominance over their bodies by walking barefoot across hot coals while the group chanted, "Cool moss. Cool moss. Cool moss."

Less dramatically shaken up by the Simonton never-never world, I readily agreed when my solemn, highly trained oncologist Philip Cohen suggested I make an appointment at Lynn Brallier's Stress Management Center. Here, I understood, I would be helped to deal not with curious theories but with real problems: the doctors had stopped giving me Adriamycin, the powerful "red devil" that had helped me so dramatically (but that can prove cardiotoxic). Bone scans and blood "markers" showed my

illness to be stable. But the more I missed the chemotherapy
that had saved my life and the more I worried lest the new
milder treatment fail, the more my bones and muscles ached
and the more concerned I grew.

At this Stress Management Center, I found a measure of pro-
fessionalism, solid training, and solid help. Lynn Brallier, Ph.D.,
a psychiatric nurse who had practiced biofeedback at the Psychiatric Institute of Washington, tried different approaches, some
"holistic," or unconventional, some not. Therapeutic touch,
wherein she passed her hands over my back (but did not touch
it), felt warm and may have shifted the energy field around my
body, but it did little for my pain. On the other hand, when she
measured my bodily responses to stress (how much I sweated
and how my temperature changed, for instance, counting back-
ward from 300 by 17s) on tricky little biofeedback machines
strapped to my hands, wrists, and head, I found I could warm my
hands and so feel more in control of my cancer-ridden body.

Somewhat to my surprise, the relaxation tapes Lynn gave me
to use two to six times a day turned out to be a smashing success. Hard-driving I, who sometimes did not even want to stop
for lunch, found myself listening to them regularly. As I heard
that calm, low voice instructing me how to relax my muscles,
from the tiny ones on my scalp down to those in every toe, tension ebbed. At night, when I turned on another Brallier tape,
Suggestions for Restful Sleep ("Say to yourself, I am at peace. I
am at peace. You are falling asleep now, you are falling asleep"),
I fell asleep—and still do.

The acupuncture chart on the wall did not bother me; I looked
forward to seeing the skillful massage therapist in an adjoining
office, who seemed to understand just how the various parts of
my creaking body fit together. After she had manipulated the
right muscles and pressed the right joints, I felt energized
instead of tired. And when Lynn—semiretired now but still
dispensing her tapes and counseling via phone and Internet—
discussed my difficulties with me or talked (unlike a traditional
psychotherapist) to my doctor or my husband about them, she
helped me stay on an even keel. She did not seem to blame me
for my cancer; indeed, she emphasized wellness, instead of ill-

ness, not what was bad with me, but what was good. I was even able to treat my second mastectomy (and third operation) as though it were another bump on a bumpy road.

I had found the sort of help that felt comfortable to me—in a place that used promising complementary treatments and was staffed by trained, credentialed people willing, even anxious, to integrate their treatments into the medical system, rather than sneer at its foibles. The Medical Illness Counseling Center in Chevy Chase, Maryland, founded by two psychiatrists, Lucy Waletzky and Stephen Hersh, was another such place.

This center is now headed solely by Hersh, author of *Beyond Miracles: Living with Cancer.* In this book, he explains that therapies resulting from systematic observations, thought, and study over meaningful periods of time—including those like radiation and chemotherapy, once considered outré—produce "measurable and repeatedly positive improvements in function and in health."

The psychiatrist agrees with the basic tenet of Western, evidence-based medicine: any competently trained responsible person with the same resources should be able to replicate research that results in such improvements and obtain positive results more than half of the time. But, he continues, unconventional health care systems have not measured the outcome of most of their work as conventional medicine has done. What's more, many of its practitioners have depended more on folk wisdom than double-blind studies in offering their products to a vulnerable public. "I have often seen nontraditional treatments be useful to patients," Hersh reports; "I have *never* seen a cure or a miracle occur in response to one of them."

That is why, when I went to the Medical Illness Counseling Center in the late 1980s, I felt I had access to the best of both mainstream and those out-of-the-mainstream mind/body or manual healing treatments that have particularly appealed to me—physiotherapy as well as biofeedback, and support from a psychiatrist committed to working with my oncologist as well as a variety of support groups.

By the 1990s, the era of Prozac, genetics, and managed care, the unconventional treatment scene had changed remarkably. On a

British trip, I read in the *Daily Telegraph* that the Prince of Wales, under fire in other ways, had made a speech championing the "alternative option" popular with the public, despite the "withering gaze of medical orthodoxy." What's more, his family all travel with a few homeopathic supplies in their medical pack, and royal doctors are all well versed in the latest complementary techniques.

In the United States the same was true: American patients, including cancer survivors, were using such therapies, not chiefly as alternatives to conventional treatment, but as supplements to it. Very few, according to the authorities, turned to controversial pharmacologic and biological Laetrile-like "cures" in lieu of conventional treatment.

And their number, as well as the amount of money being paid for services, had increased dramatically—even in the short span between 1990 and 1997. Some eighty-three million American adults—more than four out of ten—used some form of alternative medical treatment in 1997, compared with three in ten in 1990, according to two widely publicized surveys published in the *New England Journal of Medicine* and, later, the *Journal of the American Medical Association* by a research team headed by Dr. David M. Eisenberg, Harvard University professor of medicine. Patient visits to alternative therapy providers had increased by 47.3 percent in the seven years between the surveys, while the amount paid for such services had risen 45 percent—from $13.7 to $27 billion, most of it not reimbursed by insurers and so paid out of pocket.

Defining such therapies as medical interventions neither widely taught in U.S. medical schools nor generally available at U.S. hospitals (like acupuncture, herbal supplements, chiropractic and massage therapy), and extrapolating their findings to the whole population, the team amplified: although the prominence of alternative medicine increased by 25 percent between surveys, and although patient visits to alternative practitioners continued to exceed visits to all U.S. primary care physicians, the extent to which patients disclosed their use of their therapies remained (and remains) low.

The good news, in the words of Barrie Cassileth, Ph.D., a recognized authority in the field: "Most of us are wise enough not to reject the high-tech wonders of mainstream medical care when serious illness strikes." In both 1990 and 1997, the vast majority (96 percent) of those who used alternative treatments for a "principal" medical condition also saw a medical doctor.

The not-so-good news: less than 40 percent of the alternative therapies used were disclosed to physicians in both years. Perhaps people feared their doctors would scorn them, even drop them as patients, if they made such a confession. More likely, it seems to me, the short present-day visits with their doctors—part of what sociologist George Ritzer calls "The McDonaldization of Society"—probably did not leave them the time necessary to explore the issue. Whatever the reason, it was, as the Eisenberg researchers put it, "don't ask, don't tell," with a substantial portion of the therapies self-administered—without advice from either practitioner or doctor, leaving some fifteen million adults at risk for potential adverse interactions involving prescription medications and herbs or high-dose vitamin supplements.

This despite the fact that people who turned to "alternative" treatments, according to the Eisenberg team surveys, were not rare and somehow marginal—emotionally immature, perhaps, lacking in courage, or poorly educated—but people who had relatively more education and higher incomes. Most used them for chronic medical conditions—conditions such as anxiety and back problems (which might well have been the results of serious disease rather than the disease itself).

The scene had changed in other ways as well. With unconventional therapies out of the closet, and to some extent demystified, the previous decade's gurus—the Simontons, for instance—had largely moved off the cancer survivor's radar screen (though their guided imagery techniques had not). Even Bernie Siegel, the onetime Yale surgeon who held us survivors responsible for our cancers when we did not love ourselves enough, was no longer playing to packed houses for high prices.

There was more interest in the work of painstaking researchers like Stanford University psychiatrist David Spiegel, whose ten-year watershed study showed that participation in a professionally led support group not only improved the quality of life of patients with breast cancer but doubled their length of life. In his *Living beyond Limits,* Spiegel explains that the evidence seems to be pointing toward a type of intervention "facing directly the threat posed by the illness and increasing social support, rather than positive mental imagery. Facing bad possibilities does not . . . convert them into bad probabilities."

And, though they seem to enjoy a degree of commercial success, there seemed to be less interest among survivors in the older, shriller "inspirational" books, as well as in those by the current self-help high rollers Dr. Andrew Weil and the more spiritually oriented Ayurveda practitioner Dr. Deepak Chopra, who do not focus particularly on cancer. As we survivors have gained more experience and a greater measure of sophistication about gathering information and making commonsense choices, we turn to such dispassionate informational books as Michael Lerner's *Choices in Healing* and *The Alternative Medicine Handbook* by Barrie Cassileth, who makes the distinction between "popular" alternative (unproven) and "helpful" complementary (adjunctive) therapies.

But perhaps the most significant change of all had begun to take place within mainstream medicine itself—once almost impervious to patient interest in matters holistic, and even cautious about the sort of conventional psychosocial interventions pioneered by mental health professionals like Sloan-Kettering's psychiatric chief, Dr. Jimmie Holland. Not only had cancer centers and hospitals set up psycho-oncological programs or at least resources for their patients and supporters, but they had begun to include a few popular out-of-the-mainstream approaches as well (particularly relaxation techniques and visual imagery).

When a favorite former boss of mine, then Health, Education, and Welfare Secretary Wilbur J. Cohen, had an important matter to discuss, he used to tell us underlings to put everything else aside and make way for "Big Medicine." Today's twenty-seven-billion-dollar-plus complementary practices picture is big medicine indeed, and in an increasingly competitive market, the once wary health care system has begun to pay it real attention. Responding to client demand—and understandably nervous about the large portion of patients who fail to share their use of complementary treatments with their physicians—mainstream medicine has started not only to take a less condescending view toward treatments it now calls "complementary and alternative" but to "integrate" those it deems safe and at least ameliorative into its own practices, even if they have not been proved effective through rigorous, randomized, controlled studies.

As one doctor friend of mine puts it: "Medical centers may be slow, but they are not dumb." So, a Sloan-Kettering nurse on an informational Cancer Care teleconference call on pain management led the hundreds of survivors listening across the country in a relaxation session. And in September 1998, the University of Texas's M. D. Anderson Cancer Center opened Place . . . of wellness, a first of its kind, one-stop multidisciplinary service providing adjunctive therapies to cancer patients (and their caregivers) aiming to help them adjust mentally, spiritually, and physically to life after cancer.

Again, on a bulletin board of Georgetown University's Lombardi Cancer Center the other day, I read a flyer advertising "Healing the Body, Mind & Spirit," a three-level program ($75 for the first two levels, $25 for the third) offering "an alternative support as a complement to conventional cancer treatment" including:

> The practice of relaxation through meditation and breathing awareness (silent mind, peaceful body);
> The nature of healing energy, discovering our centers of perception (Yin and Yang);
> The release of stress through centering and movement awareness (Yoga and Tai-Chi);
> The opening of the heart, the power of prayer through visualization and affirmation (Healing Energy).

Beyond such offerings, we find conferences and workshops in unconventional medicine at major universities, with some 43 of the 125 American medical schools offering courses ranging from "Chinese QiGong I & II" (Case Western Reserve University School of Medicine) to "Complementary Medicine," an integrated first-, second-, and fourth-year program (Cornell Medical

College). On the practical side, a growing number of insurers are giving members a choice of complementary services.

What's more, the federal government has become much more involved. In October 1998, President Clinton signed a law upgrading the Office of Alternative Medicine (established in 1991) at the National Institutes of Health into the National Center for Complementary and Alternative Medicine, with an annual budget of $50 million, increased from $20 million. Since 60 to 70 percent of the calls that come into this office's information clearinghouse are cancer calls, it is good to know that the center will intensify its efforts to evaluate complementary and alternative medical treatments and hold them up to rigorous scientific standards. In the same way it was good to read that the American Medical Association planned to publish some eighty reports on various alternative therapies in its own and other scientific journals, some involving randomized controlled clinical trials (a crucial research step largely missing on the alternative scene since the trials that put the use of the apricot seed derivative Laetrile to rest at the end of the 1970s).

At least one widely used out-of-the-mainstream treatment—acupuncture—has been recommended as effective for certain uses (including postoperative and chemotherapy nausea and vomiting) by a consensus panel convened by the National Institutes of Health. What's more, the Food and Drug Administration has allowed acupuncture needles to be used generally as a legitimate medical device.

I know I have been lucky; I have enjoyed excellent care and have not needed to dream of miracles and spontaneous remissions that occasionally do occur, with or without any kind of treatment. I have been able to gain a measure of serenity from therapies like massage or yoga without wondering if I was undergoing a "placebo effect."

When rookie survivors ask me for advice about unconventional treatments, as they frequently do, I fantasize about creating a tape for them, in which one side of me (TS—The Skeptic) would chat with the other (W,M—Well, Maybe). This is how the dialogue would go:

TS: The longer I hang in, the more experience I gain, the less I can imagine using a nonmainstream treatment as an alternative rather than a supplement. I could *never* imagine using one of the unproven pharmacologic and biologic treatments like Dr. Stanislaw Burzynski's Antineoplaston treatment (using synthesized urine proteins), which remains in demand in his Texas clinic despite serious legal troubles. Or shark cartilage, which survivors used to think had an antitumor effect but which a study reported in a 1998 issue of the *Journal of Clinical Oncology* proved "inactive in patients with advanced-stage cancer and no salutary effect on quality of life."

  Nor could I imagine taking a coffee enema in a south-of-the-border clinic, no matter how cleansing or purifying (too much caffeine upsets me from the top; common sense tells me not to try it from the bottom).

W,M: But you did try acupuncture, when your internist recommended a credentialed practitioner who he knew would use clean needles. Perhaps you did not give it enough of a try; you wanted a quick fix like most Americans. . . .

TS: His needles produced a nice warm temporary glow when they were inserted into my back and chest, but they didn't take away the pain. And the treatment seemed pricey for what I got out of it; substantial charges you've got to pay out of your own pocket are hardly a trivial issue.

W,M: You're right. Still, we survivors have to deal with this crazy disease, creeping around slyly inside of us. It's no wonder we look for folk treatments we know benefited ancient societies. Or "natural" therapies derived from plants and trees—treatments that seem less harsh than those that make your hair fall out and your stomach churn.

TS: That nonmainstream "natural" versus mainstream "unnatural" argument impresses me not. Which is which? Is the drug penicillin, which came from molds, not natural? And wasn't I once almost killed by the "natural" effects of a poisonous snake bite? Haven't I seen people close to me laid low by poison ivy and poison oak (though fortunately, not

poisonous mushrooms)? And I cannot knock the tough
chemo (derived, at times, from tree barks and the like),
which turned my disease around so dramatically; really, it
was a quid pro quo—harsh treatment in exchange for years of
lovely life.

W,M: When you cook, you use a lot of "natural" herbs.

TS: As flavoring. But not as medicine. Some of the herbs survivors take may be harmless, but not others. The Food and
Drug Administration, which, under an unfortunate law, cannot apply the same strict regulation to dietary substances
(including herbs used for medicinal purposes) that it applies
to drugs, has been especially concerned about herbal remedies containing the "upper" or stimulant ephedrine, which
can cause serious side effects and even death.

And my oncologist worries about the presence of active
and potentially toxic substances like arsenic in Chinese folk
medicine now being used for certain types of leukemia.

W,M: Couldn't you just warn rookie survivor friends, *Caveat Emptor,* which for the Latin-challenged means "Let the Buyer
Beware"? After all, we survivors could all learn, with the
help of those authoritative, user-friendly books you rely on,
to be realistic about the level of our expectations. We could
learn to separate empty unproven promises from solid helpful proven therapies.

TS: One can stumble, confused, among the promises. As Barrie
Cassileth points out, a remedy like aromatherapy can be
pleasant and calming when it is used as a soothing fragrance
in the bath or during massage, but used as a cure for disease
(which some proponents claim), it could delay needed conventional treatment and so prove harmful.

W,M: How about mind/body therapies? They don't do you or your
pocketbook much harm when they're used as a complement
to mainstream treatment. Meditation—massage—those sort of
treatments make a lot of us feel so relaxed—so *good.*

TS: True. When the practitioner is properly trained and licensed,
such help can give you a measure of peace and serenity. But

you cannot always do what makes you feel good. I sat in the sun baking my skin for years and felt wonderful; now, my dermatologists say, I'm paying the price in skin cancers.

W,M: Still, you've profited from some of the nonmainstream mind-body treatments that are based on the notion that you can influence the course of your disease instead of lying back, victimlike, and letting it walk all over you. The theory is that long-term stress can depress the immune system, that positive emotions strengthen it, and that a strengthened immune system makes the possibility of fighting off cancer more likely.

TS: That's the theory. I'm wary of theories that have not been conclusively proved (one medical scientist calls them "puta-tive"). And I'm wary of alternative/complementary true believers who lead survivors up the garden path touting research that seems to confirm their promises and omitting others that do not confirm them.

W,M: Wary is as wary does. It's true, isn't it, that long-term stres-sors can nag at us and affect our bodies? I reviewed a book with a cute title: *Why Zebras Don't Get Ulcers.* According to the neuroscientist-author, animals have the same physical responses to stress that we do—the body mobilizes its resources to survive, enabling the heart to pound faster, the blood pressure to rise, and the breathing rate to increase so we can fight or flee.

This matters little in the short run. But long-term stres-sors (like worries about your next mortgage payment or an uncomfortable marriage or an unappreciative boss) unknown to zebras can nag us human beings until they create bodily uproars that last for months—and eventually can make you sick.

TS: Indeed, as the old ditty goes, a person can develop a cold, and other miseries as well, as a result of stress (though doctors now treat some ulcers—once popularly considered very stress-related—successfully with antibacterial medicines). But bioscientists I respect say you cannot really compare the role the immune system plays in fighting off infectious diseases like the common cold with the complex role it might play in slow-growing cancers.

What's more, you cannot always apply to complicated human beings what you learn from studying animals. All the variables are easier to control in animals, and they can often be productively observed in ten days instead of ten years and even sacrificed in the cause of research (to examine tissue, for example).

W,M: Yet long-term stress might play a role?

TS: We don't really know yet. There's data to suggest psychological influences on the immune system, but we don't know if that is powerful enough to affect the development and/or progression of cancer (the mechanisms might be different). Right now, some say it looks as though the effect is minimal. Others believe the data is just not there; the exact connection between cortical function and bodily response in cancer is still largely speculative.

W,M: Look, mainstream medicine *does* support, even encourage, psychosocial interventions that help us, not to stay absolutely stress-free (that's impossible), but to control the stress we encounter in the normal course of living and so improve our quality of life.

TS: You've got it: to improve our quality of life. But at this early stage, medical science does not know precisely what such interventions can accomplish.

W,M: Too complicated for me.

TS: For most of us survivors. There's now a voluminous research literature—including animal and clinical studies—examining the role of the immune system in cancer. Dr. Dana Bovbjerg, a—get this—psychoneuroimmunologist at New York's Mount Sinai Medical Center, says this has been called a literature of "great expectations and bitter disappointments." Even with the simpler models provided by animal research, results can be contradictory: stress some mice, and they fall victim to cancer; stress others, and their resistance improves. This does not mean the mind-body cancer connection through the immune system does not exist. But the evidence is controversial; we need more of it.

W,M: Sloan-Kettering's Dr. Jimmie Holland says studies indicating that psychological interventions might enhance the human immune system and so play a role in either cancer incidence or progression are "blips on the screen."

TS: Dr. Bovbjerg feels there's not enough information out there on the screen even to use the word *blips.* In a chapter prepared for the second edition of *The Handbook of Psycho-oncology* (now titled *Textbook of Psycho-Oncology*), he points out that "naturalistic studies" of people (in their daily lives rather than in the laboratory) facing a variety of life "stressors," such as academic examinations, surviving the death of a spouse, even living close to Three Mile Island or having a partner undergo a bone marrow transplant, have consistently found changes in a number of measures of immune function (decreased "natural killer," or NK cell activity, for instance).

But such studies do not examine the responsible mechanisms. The same could be said of a number of psychosocial studies featuring intervention techniques like relaxation or biofeedback.

W,M: Whatever cooks with all those NK or T cells (suppressor or other cells that interact with each other and with our organs), experts and survivors everywhere were excited about the possibilities raised by the ten-year mind-body study at Stanford University done by psychiatrist David Spiegel, M.D. This showed that participation in a professionally led support group not only improved the quality of life of patients with metastatic breast cancer but doubled their length of life.

And a study of melanoma patients by UCLA's Fawzy Fawzy, M.D., concluded that a more limited psychological intervention had results similar to Spiegel's—not only lowering depression, fatigue, and the like but also affecting immune functions and lengthening survival time. Probably as a result of these studies, group therapy with other survivors is now recommended more often as part of a cancer treatment regimen, according to psychiatrist Stephen Hersh, especially in the first year after diagnosis.

TS: Still, replication of the studies has been slow in coming, and in a gracious editorial accompanying publication of the results of a study conducted among a large number of women with stage II breast cancer, of the relationship between psychological distress and survival, Spiegel himself concluded: "There is little in the present data to encourage even the most optimistic advocates of the connection between psychosocial and medical variables."

W,M: Hey! As a cancer survivor, I *want* to believe that our attitude—what the scientists call our "fighting spirit"—has an effect on the length as well as the quality of our lives!

TS: I do too. But only if survivors do not feel guilty if that fighting spirit proves ineffective. We do not cause our cancers, or recurrence of our cancers. *We do not.* A host of factors—like our genetic makeup or the way our hormonal system functions—all strongly affect what happens to us, cancerwise. The big predictors for recurrence are not your emotional or psychological state, the experts say, but the medical variables you would suspect (like how many positive nodes you have in breast cancer).

W,M: As Dr. Spiegel puts it, for survivors "it is not simply mind over matter" but instead how to fashion future research so that "it may be possible to determine how mind does matter."

TS: Amen.

8 ❧ *Significant Others*
A Part of the Main

> No man is an *Iland*, intire of it selfe; every man is a peece of
> the *Continent*, a part of the *maine*; if a *Clod* bee washed away
> by the *Sea, Europe* is the lesse, as well as if a *Promontorie*
> were, as well as if a *Mannor* of thy *friends* or of *thine owne*
> were; any mans *death* diminishes *me,* because I am involved
> in *Mankinde;* And therefore never send to know for whom
> the *bell* tolls; It tolls for *thee.*
> —John Donne, Meditation XVII

No one knows better than the cancer survivor that no man or
woman is an island, entire of itself. No one knows better than
the survivor, no matter what phase of the journey he or she is
traveling, that each of us is a piece of the continent, a part of the
main. The bell signaling involvement in humankind tolls for the
cancer survivor with singular force and intensity.

This is because we who have endured sometimes extended,
sometimes shorter, but still esoteric and often debilitating treatment in exchange for life become more keenly aware of the way
our lives intertwine with others as every month and every year
passes. The French have a saying that translates: "to say goodbye
is to die a little." We hope our deaths will diminish those who
outlive us, at least a little. Meanwhile, our continued involvement with those we value—our families, close friends, any of the
human beings whom the therapists have antiseptically dubbed
"significant others"—increases our ability to handle serious illness and its consequences.

As cancer has become more of a long-term, chronic disease, instead of a temporary crisis from which we emerge triumphantly "cured" or not at all, our bonds with other people continue to buttress our lives. This does not mean they cannot and do not change. Bonds with those we care for, and who care for us, can grow stronger, while bonds with others can weaken, even break—perhaps because they cannot accept us as we have become, or vice versa.

And as we survivors have grown more independent, more recognized, not as victims but as functioning people able to speak and act for ourselves, our ability to influence the way we live with other people has increased. We now know we do not need to retire from the world and its activities. Instead, we can adapt to it and learn to lead "A Different Kind of Life," as a public television show I participated in was titled—a life limited, perhaps, by the effects of illness but which we approach alive and kicking.

Appearing on this TV program in the early 1980s, my husband, Jerry, explained what this different life with me was like at that intermediate stage of my journey. He reported that as we left the beach cottage we loved on the Delaware shore each Labor Day weekend, I mused, as I never had before, "I wonder if I'll ever see this place again."

He added that, living with me, he sometimes felt like the ground crew for a supersonic plane: off and flying I traveled at top speed, but when I landed (often flat on my bed upstairs at 5:30 P.M.), I needed a certain amount of service between flights. My energy was limited, and he needed to do many things that I used to do (like washing the dinner dishes) so I would have the strength to do what I want.

More than a decade later, I still crave independence, but I know I am invariably dependent on other people, though perhaps in different ways. As I and others have become more seasoned survivors (and our families with us), we have learned that total independence is impossible. Our often can-do culture's emphasis on independence might make this seem wrong, even bad, but it is not.

On the contrary, some dependency, a positive dependency, or interdependency that recognizes the limits of survivorship may be a sign of maturity and of a pragmatic willingness to accept our situation. Now, for example, my worries about our still beloved beach cottage have shifted: I now worry, not about dying before I can see it again (though that may happen!), but about whether keeping it up and regularly driving long distances down to the shore and back have become too much for me—and my husband. So we have started to rent the house more and make less demanding summer plans.

I seldom meet survivors anymore who refuse to make the switch from living as a "sick" person to living as a "different" one, who (theoretically) are satisfying some sort of "secondary gains" or unconscious needs—to behave as a child, stay home from a dull job, curl up in bed, be the center of attention, and get taken care of. On the contrary, the vast majority of the survivors I know try, sometimes against great odds, to gain all possible independence and freedom of choice and live as responsible adults in the adult world.

And we want our families, our friends, and even our acquaintances to see us that way. When I prepared the Cancer Survivors' Bill of Rights in 1988, I was surprised at the warmth with which my peers received it—and still do; one survivor colleague, saying it had "taken on a wonderful life of its own," takes it with him on all his speaking tours. I was surprised, too, that the sections seemingly most appreciated had to do, not as much with important practical topics like equal job opportunity, health insurance coverage, and the assurance of needed lifelong medical care, as with our right to the pursuit of happiness in our personal lives.

This means having the right, for example, to talk with our families and friends about our cancer experience if we wish, but to refuse to discuss it if that is our choice, and not to be expected to be more upbeat or less blue than anyone else. And it means the right to be free of the stigma of cancer as a "dread disease" in all social relations, and of blame for having gotten the disease and having survived it.

I am now no longer surprised at the importance of this sort of personal theme for cancer survivors. I know full well how deeply we yearn for self-esteem and dignity in dealing with others. I know, too, that our special message is that though our distinctive needs must be met, our feelings as members of the human family cannot be ignored.

Family! No doubt about it, the nature of this embattled entity has changed in the past decades as much as the nature of cancer itself and the nature of its survivors. With almost half of new marriages ending in divorce, men and women experimenting with all sorts of novel living arrangements, and children conceived in petri dishes growing up shuttling between households and then taking off for college and adult lives in scattered places, it is no longer possible for the horse to know the way to carry the sleigh. Even should that sleigh arrive successfully at grandmother's house, that lady may be off pursuing pleasures undreamed of in generations past, and unavailable for hosting holiday dinners.

No matter. However you define the family, it is where we find the most significant of the others in our lives, the people we care for and depend on—as they depend on us. This family may still be composed of a husband, wife, and pair of children (with a grandparent living happily around the corner and available for baby-sitting and other support). Or it may be like the "Funny Family" I first read about in the *Washington Post*'s Style section a few years ago. This was a group of a dozen friends who organized at the request of a divorced mother of two teenage girls, prodded by her therapist.

Pooling their resources, they undertook specific tasks and assignments—grocery shopping, cooking and cleaning as a team, accompanying the patient from doctor to doctor and test to test, filling out insurance forms, even organizing her daughter's wedding. Astonished at the power of their group—which in the heat of battle truly became Shakespeare's "few, we happy few, we band of brothers"—they wrote a no-nonsense book for caretakers (*Share the Care: How to Organize a Group to Care for Someone Who Is Seriously Ill*). This enlightening guide recognizes some unromantic realities: sick people can complain, caretakers can be control freaks, and everyone should get to be boss, but not for too long.

More and more, cancer is regarded as a family affair. From the beginning, we survivors usually turn to our families—however

they be composed—for refuge and support. The world may be, as
the poet put it, a "darkling plain, swept with confused alarm of
struggle and flight, where ignorant armies clash by night," but at
home we hope to find a measure of certitude and peace, as well
as help for pain.

The other side of the late-twentieth-century coin is the
increased recognition that family members can be deeply and
poignantly affected by the disease of one of their members. They
can be viewed, suggests Sloan-Kettering psychiatrist Marguerite
S. Lederberg, as "second order patients," or survivors in their
own right. In fact, they are accepted as such as members of the
National Coalition for Cancer Survivorship (NCCS). And the
Springfield, Missouri members of Make Today Count, one of the
older cancer survivor organizations, recently issued an updated
version of its Bill of Rights, beginning: "It is my right to honor
my own needs. When I take care of myself I am able to give the
best care and attention to the patient."

If the tone of this document is somewhat more petulant than
that of the earlier bill I drafted for survivors themselves (stipu-
lating, for example, "It is my right to have my own feelings. I am
having a tough time too"), it is possibly because of the onerous
caretaking burden many have been forced to assume in an era of
"managed care." With hospitals dismissing patients earlier and
earlier, it's not at all unusual for families to have to supervise
complex medical regimens—tube feedings, for example, or
chemotherapy administered through intravenous lines.

In Western cultures, the period when patients were taken care of
in hospitals may turn out to be "a brief aberration in social and
medical history," as family expert and psychiatrist Marguerite
Lederberg has put it. Now, in developed countries, political and
financial considerations are conspiring to return patients home
at a rapidly increasing rate; the home, however comfortable and
suitable, is the locus of care as it was long ago (and still is in less
developed cultures). Relatives and friends usually rally round,
doing their best, and indeed, they often show great nobility and
strength. But difficult caretaking situations may last for long
periods, and the emotional—as well as financial and social—cost

may be high, with savings accounts drained and careers held back or, at least, put on hold.

Reviewing the burgeoning literature on the contributions families make to patient care in her chapter of the new edition of *Psycho-Oncology*, Dr. Lederberg leads her list with the provision of *emotional* support. No wonder. Often, as I have watched a couple holding hands—he almost in tears, she tense and stoic—in a physician's office, waiting for the results of her difficult biopsy, I have thought how differently family members support each other. Pairs like this leave me with quite a different feeling than did a recently remarried lawyer with breast surgery I once met in a health club dressing room after a swim: her husband and five children, who ranged in age from twelve to twenty, were a little more solicitous, perhaps, than they used to be—the younger children touched her a bit more to make sure she was there; a twenty-year-old son called from another city to play her special guitar music, while a teenage daughter, whom she had taught to examine her own breasts, joked, "Mom, how are you and your new boob?" Each behaved independently, coolly, and cheerfully as they did their own thing, pitching in and taking care of each other.

If emotional support can be offered with good humor and cheer, and without criticism, that's appreciated. But the best support is that tailored to meet the individual survivor's needs. One husband I knew well did a heroic job taking care of his wife while she lay abed for months with a cruel brain tumor that demolished her sense of self. He did not seem to realize he expected too much from her, including a brave front before their multitude of friends as well as deep intimate discussions about the meaning of life and death, when she would have preferred being left alone to relax watching old-time TV comedies.

Information (along with *Shared Responsibility for Decision Making*), the second family contribution on the Lederberg list, must also be tailored for the individual survivor. As word of new or more effective life-extending and pain-easing treatments spreads, family members can grow as hungry for it as survivors themselves. Indeed, they often take on the bulk of the information seeking, and some survivors are happy to relinquish this

time-consuming task—particularly in the early stages of an illness. But later on, as they feel less helpless, they may achieve
more sense of control by doing most of their own research and
participating in their own decision making with their medical
teams.

At first, I know I depended a good deal on my brother, a Baltimore psychiatrist, to talk to my doctors, to glean information,
and help with decision making. But as the years have passed, and
as I've gained confidence and learned my way in the medical
system, I've not needed my brother or other knowledgeable
friends to mediate for me. To put this another way, in one recent
week, I heard from three friends (a solicitous sister, a business-
like father, and a worried mother-in-law) each seeking news
about treatment options for a survivor. I sensed that the help of
the first two was indispensable, while that of the third, though
useful, seemed stereotypically mother-in-lawish and—well—
dispensable to the survivor.

The next family contributions in line on the Lederberg list—
Concrete Caregiving and *Meeting Financial and Social Costs*—
are self-evident (and staggering, with as many as a quarter of
primary caregivers giving up or losing their jobs, and one-third
of families losing all their savings or major source of income).
But whether the subject at hand is something as sensitive as a
needed switch in family roles—related to parenting or home-
making or breadwinning—or as mundane as continuing to perform standard family functions, the family must help *Maintain
Stability* and, at the same time, *Adapt to Change.*

Change may be the only constant, since survivors' needs differ so markedly. Most of the social scientists who have studied
cancer families seem to feel that communication between their
individual members is crucial in avoiding conflict. Psychiatrist
Stephen Hersh even suggests the survivor take the lead early on,
calling a meeting (or "news conference") of family members and
close friends to discuss what lies ahead—from who is going to
walk the dog or act as family chauffeur to how to handle repeti-
tive medical condition questions ("how is she doing—really?").

But Mills College sociologist Laura E. Nathan, one of the
newer researchers who have helped focus attention on families

dealing with the uncertainties of long-term survivorship, points out that such a blatant approach may not always be best. Although the bulk of the literature on communication in the family emphasizes the benefits of open communication (since it helps ease stress and overall adaptation), she reports that there is evidence that, for some, avoiding discussion of the cancer and its accompanying threat may be a "positive coping mechanism."

I agree. It does no harm to keep pointing out that different survivors, like other people, have different needs. One size seldom fits all: letting it all hang out within the family may suit some, particularly younger people, and provide them with better understanding as well as a temporary catharsis. But I have found that when you deal with close-to-the-heart chronic cancer matters—like the seemingly foolish anxiety, even terror, that comes with the end of bouts of treatment, or the never-ending, nagging fear of recurrence, it may be better to play your cards a bit closer to your chest and turn outside the family for professional help.

One divorced friend of mine, for instance, sensed that she was leaning on an older son in inappropriate ways (asking him to rub her back, for instance). She found a competent counselor (and through him, a massage therapist) to help her over the bumps. Another survivor was not so lucky. When I heard that her husband had vanished after his wife's mastectomy, I reacted strongly: "She's better off without him!" But the bearer of the tale had a different view: "It's a bullshit society!"

Spouses, experts agree, are generally, and naturally, the hardest hit by a cancer experience. Sometimes they show levels of emotional and functional disruption as great as or greater than that of the patient—and these worsen with time, independent of patient mood or health. Male spouses feel more distressed than female, but when men become patients, they are less depressed. As for mastectomy spouses, a study found them to be deeply emotionally engaged but hiding it and minimizing in a way they thought was supportive.

Listening in (with some 499 other women and men) on a Cancer Care teleconference call entitled "Living beyond Breast Cancer: Intimacy, Sexuality, and Love," I marveled at the way the old tendency to romanticize the problems surrounding sex is giving way to hard-nosed realism. Led by Marisa Weiss, M.D., author of *Living beyond Breast Cancer* and founder of a Pennsylvania-based organization with that name, the group energetically and explicitly addressed problems and fears—like loss of sexual attractiveness, painful intercourse, and discomfort at having your body seen nude after surgery.

When one woman reported with infinite sadness in her voice that she and her husband had not even been able to speak to each other about sex since her surgery, the social worker in charge of the call volunteered to call her personally after the conference call to discuss the matter. That this questioner is not alone is seen in a Living Beyond Breast Cancer survey showing that most (63 percent) of some 284 breast cancer survivors wanted to discuss sexuality with their caregivers yet few (15 percent) had ever done so even if they were willing to initiate the discussion themselves. The women with the most significant problems were the least likely to have had this discussion.

Open communication seems to work best with another group of survivor family members who need special help: children of parents with cancer. The child who sees Mom or Dad at home in bed, gone from the house for treatment, or simply changed in appearance understandably becomes anxious. Such children can show various psychological symptoms and acting-out behaviors, developing school problems and even long-term changes in cognitive performance and personality (such as self-esteem). Even if they have simply taken to lounging helplessly around the house, these children experience guilt about the possibility that they caused this mysterious illness, fear for themselves, and grief and yearning for lost parenting.

But it does not have to be that way. Dr. Wendy Harpham, the mother of three little children when she developed non-Hodgkin's lymphoma, has shown that. In her book *When a Parent Has Cancer* (and its companion book for kids, *Becky and the Worry Cup*), Wendy explains that the greatest gift one can give to children is not protection from stress, change, or loss but the confidence and tools to cope with and grow with all that life offers, both the good and the bad.

Her suggestions agree with those of other experts: tell your children the truth, for they must always be able to trust you. Reassure them that they will be cared for, no matter what happens. Take care of your own needs, for nothing is more important to your children than your getting well. Realize that you can teach a lot about life and caring in a little time. And a theme that runs through all the literature for survivorship families—get help when you need it.

Not only did Wendy raise her children in a life-affirming way after she developed cancer, but she also used her gift for writing to pass that affirmation on to other parent/survivors. I have always felt that she, like others who have gone on to marry and have children despite the uncertainties of the hanging-in life, personifies the ultimate in survivorship. Another of this spunky crew is Andrea DiLorenzo, a soft-spoken policy analyst for the National Education Association in her mid-forties, who seems to be totally in charge of her life.

Andrea, whose husband proposed to her after her first breast cancer surgery but before treatment for ovarian cancer, looks back at her second recurrence (a second breast primary and third cancer) and remembers the thought of getting back into the medical system and undergoing treatment again as a "horror." But she did it; this time, she chose a mastectomy with a silicone implant and prefers the results to her lumpectomy, which she refers to as "a wounded breast." Now, after fourteen years as a survivor, she and her husband have adopted two Brazilian children—a seven-year-old boy and ten-year-old girl. Ola!

Scientists use the word *homeostasis* to describe the process whereby the human body tries to maintain a steady state in the face of environmental change. Take a change in temperature. If you jog in the sun and get too hot and uncomfortable, your skin senses this and sends a message to your brain. You perspire, getting rid of heat. You also probably stop jogging and move into the shade to rest. In the same way that individuals adapt to change, the family unit senses change and tries in conscious and unconscious ways to maintain its internal balance.

The first differences are obvious: families, like individuals, find themselves at different ages and stages of development when illness strikes. Young people, just starting careers and families, find themselves behind a different eight ball than middle-aged folk who have established family "launching centers" (with their first or even last child gone). Probably unused to being sick, they have less financial and job security. Sadly, their paths are blocked just as they are starting out.

Middle-aged families have another set of problems. With their children gone, with their own parents becoming ill or dependent, perhaps demanding attention in their own homes or some sort of retirement community, they may have been trying to establish new interests, even new careers. Illness now drains their energy and keeps them from a fresh start. They react in a different way than the young family whose nine-year-old daughter develops a nervous tic and cough when her mother's cancer metastasizes. They react in a different way, too, from the aging family already dealing with failing eyesight and hearing, memory loss, and/or bothersome joint and bone pains.

Family researchers have outdone themselves trying to characterize their subjects. They divide them into motor and cerebral groups, into open and closed systems, into mother- or father- or child-centered units, constricted, internalized, object-focused, impulsive, childlike, or chaotic types. Such classifications emphasizing maladaptive tendencies can leave the survivor a bit confused and sad.

Less jargonistic ways of thinking about the effect of cancer on families make more sense to me—more in tune with Ogden Nash's classic, very human (if dated!) definition: "A family is a unit composed not only of children, but of men, women, an occasional animal and the common cold." Or even retired Medical College of Virginia oncologist Dr. Susan Mellette's candid description of the family that denies the cancer and becomes *overdependent* on the survivor, expecting the usual, or even the impossible, of him or her. One such husband brought his lady friend to his wife's hospital bedside, expecting them to be polite to each other.

Analyzing families who are, as she puts it, in the process of adapting not to the acute phase of cancer, and not to terminal disease, "but to uncertainty," Mills College sociologist Laura E. Nathan seems to pull such concepts together in ways that make sense to seasoned, long-term survivors like me. In this social science model Nathan recognizes, and even stresses, that families do not suffer illness in a vacuum. It's true: family members are what they are; they differ greatly, just as their cancers differ; they have been behaving in certain ways, sometimes for a very long while; cancer only intensifies what was there before.

Nevertheless, the sociologist feels you can get a good idea of how they are going to adapt to the uncertain hanging-in life by considering four different "background variables": *personality and psychological* (what is their level of self-esteem and self-mastery?); *social structural and demographic* (how about educational and occupational and socioeconomic status? race and ethnicity?); *roles and relationship* (marital status? breadwinning and parenting roles?); and *disease related* (type and stage of cancer and treatment for it).

These variables affect how a family adapts directly in obvious ways: if the cancer survivor is a married, heavily involved parent, his wife and children relate differently to him than those who care for the single, childless survivor. Or if the well-off survivor suffers first-stage, almost always easily treated breast cancer, her family is in a different position than the needy survivor who is hit with metastatic lung disease.

But, as Nathan points out, these variables affect a family indirectly in less obvious ways, through distinct "coping strategies." Some, for example, use a *direct/action-oriented* style, which fully recognizes the situation and seeks to address that reality. I myself—possibly because of the way I'm wired psychologically (and perhaps because of my experience in the sociomedical culture)—have adopted the model's first "direct/action-oriented" strategy from the beginning of my cancer journey.

This has worked for me and my family. In fact, when my son Jonathan developed Hodgkin's disease a decade ago, I was pleased to see it work for him, too, as he set about collecting information, getting second and third opinions, and then organizing a smoothly functioning support system among his many friends in Atlanta. Since he was younger when cancer struck, he seemed understandably angrier than I had been—and though that felt uncomfortable to us all at times, I admired the way he was able to express his feelings and deal with them.

When Ava Fierst, a happily married thirty-six-year-old living in Massachusetts's "Happy (Connecticut River) Valley," developed an aggressive form of breast cancer a decade ago, she adopted another of Nathan's positive coping strategies, *conscious normalcy.* After her two-year-old daughter came up and slapped her as she lay in a postchemotherapy stupor on the couch, Ava decided that her illness simply could not interfere with her family's life.

Acknowledging the reality of the situation, she chose to put it to the side and continue life to the greatest extent possible. She set the tone, trying to rest when her three small children were at school and to get all the emotional and practical help she needed. One friend organized others so that in a bad six-week period the family never had to cook an evening meal. And when her lawyer husband, Fred, pitched in, "putting on armor" to assume a protective, if fighting, anticancer stance, she warned him not to handle her with "velvet gloves." She found a different sort of support from her sister-in-law, who encouraged her to go ahead remodeling her house and, eventually, to begin work toward a degree at Smith College in art history. A strong family, the Fiersts learned to live the way Ava wanted to live— "normally."

Another of Nathan's coping strategies, a *denial/suppression* mode—in which family members can deny the cancer completely, suppress their feelings about it, or simply keep distracted from the real issues—leaves something to be desired but is not always a completely negative stance (see chapter 3). An older mother, for instance, wrote to me sadly about the guilt she felt because her grown daughter, artistic and successful in public service work in a small town, had been in "total denial" of her thyroid cancer and so had not obtained the best possible treatment in time. Perhaps if these parents had understood what there was in their daughter's personality and/or social situation that caused her to adopt—in this case—such a negative coping strategy, they could have worked with her and helped her deal with her situation realistically. And they might not have lost her.

Finally, Nathan lists the almost always negative *escapist* strategy, in which the realities of cancer are avoided through the use of drugs and/or alcohol. This strategy may help for any given day, but in terms of long-term adaptation, it is not usually productive.

But in the introduction to her late husband Raymond Carver's *A New Path to the Waterfall,* writer Tess Gallagher tells us how this talented writer/survivor employed such an "escapist" strategy. In his compelling poem "Gravy," she explains, Carver in effect used his coming death from lung cancer as "proof" of a *former* escape from the death by alcoholism he narrowly avoided:

> No other word will do. For that's what it was. Gravy.
> Gravy, these past ten years.
> Alive, sober, working, loving and
> being loved by a good woman. Eleven years
> ago he was told he had six months to live
> at the rate he was going. And he was going
> nowhere but down. So he changed his ways
> somehow. He quit drinking! And the rest?
> After that it was *all* gravy, every minute
> of it, up to and including when he was told about,
> well, some things that were breaking down and
> building up inside his head. "Don't weep for me,"
> he said to his friends. "I'm a lucky man.
> I've had ten years longer than I or anyone
> expected. Pure gravy. And don't forget it."

And how do the "background variables" affect the coping styles and so the outcomes when cancer strikes minority American families—be they African American, Hispanic, Native American, Asian, Eskimo, Pacific Islander, or those just plain poor and rural? I've learned a great deal about this poignant sociocultural reality at the "Biennial Symposia on Minorities, the Medically Underserved, and Cancer," honchoed by my NCCS colleague Lovell Jones, Ph.D., of the M. D. Anderson

Cancer Center. Early on, Lovell told me his African American schoolteacher mother, who was not low-income, waited until she had a massive lump before she went for care. Why did she wait? "Because of the fear [prevalent in her culture]. She was afraid of the idea of going in. She thought a diagnosis of cancer meant automatic death."

At the 1997 symposium, another colleague, Bobbi de Cordová-Hanks, who heads Bosom Buddies, a breast cancer support and education program headquartered in Jacksonville, Florida, said Hispanic survivors have trouble making themselves understood in a medical system that values time and money and often fails to respect a culture in which a certain amount of pain and martyrdom is valued. According to Bobbi, who says she has earned her "minority" status as a Sephardic Jewish woman-over-sixty breast cancer survivor, people with a Puerto Rican background are used to going to the doctor en masse (a thirty-five-member family can show up for a medical interview). They usually pick either an older family head or a youngster fluent in English to speak for them. The problem: he or she may not really represent the patient.

And she told of a group of Russian women paralyzed when they were asked to take part in a mammography screening program. No one could understand why all these women refused to participate until she pointed out they had the "incredible fear of radiation . . . they looked at the pictures of the big machine which would look into their breasts and thought of Chernobyl."

More cultural vignettes from the 1997 symposium: a coal miner's daughter with a Ph.D. spoke, like Bobbi, of the stoicism, the "making the best of a difficult situation" attitude characteristic of Appalachian culture. On the other hand, these Appalachians have a real "sense of place" that leads them to tell cancer caregivers, "We've organized . . . we'll do it for ourselves, thank you very much."

Another Ph.D., a Native American from the Wailaki tribe in northern California who lost a leg to cancer, confessed, "My mother truly believes she was the reason I got cancer." Because of these guilt feelings, the two of them cannot talk about her cancer. Different attitudes toward time also influence the way members of her small tribe deal with cancer; for instance, its members have trouble understanding why they should stop smoking to prevent the disease because they live more in the present than in the future.

And a San Franciscan spoke of the fatalism and "inwardness" of Asian families in the face of cancer. His parents went along with his sister's tumor treatment, but could they discuss it? Not really.

Of course, while such attitudes prevail in older generations who may not have been born in the United States, they may be less apparent in the younger families born and bred here. Still, they can have a profound effect. Cancer stigma dies hard, whether within families or out in the larger society, as we will see when we explore cancer as metaphor and survivor issues in the workplace. Sometimes it can involve economic as well as emotional grief.

Family ties can express themselves in ways you never would have expected before becoming a cancer survivor.

My grandmother, Linda Miller, a brilliant (though modest) art collector, philanthropist, and talented (though unpublished) storyteller, developed cancer in the same year of her life and in the same breast as I did. We even went to the same hospital, Sloan-Kettering, located in her time on the west side of Manhattan. The difference: she lived only a bit over two years, while I have survived now for almost twenty-five.

Medical progress enhanced my chances, of course. When I speak to medical establishment audiences, I always point out that I probably had better surgery, more precise radiation, and powerful chemo and hormone therapy not available to my grandmother. Another difference: as a well-brought-up daughter of her times, she hid her disease, fleeing to Tucson, Arizona, with a niece to study at the university; she even hid her recurrence when she first felt the new tumor in her abdomen. The two hurried home to a New York hotel, checking in secretly so as not to worry my mother, while I, for better or worse—I dare to think for better—have dealt with my cancer episodes openly, if not blatantly, Oprah-style.

Cancer skipped my mother (and her sister, who died at twenty-nine of a virulent sinus infection before the days of antibiotics). My younger brother, thus far, is also cancer-free. But my two sisters developed breast cancer: Ellen beat it in her late forties only to die fifteen years later of lethal pancreatic cancer; Wendy developed the disease in her sixties—in a time when it could be caught very early on a routine mammogram and finished off with lumpectomy, radiation, and tamoxifen. For such cases, the survival rate is *very* good—as high as 96.8 percent.

When the genetic revolution arrived full blown in the 1990s and cancer genes began to be identified with startling rapidity, I simply assumed I carried some BRCA1 or BRCA2 mutation (an alteration in the gene that can interfere with proper body functions by causing the gene to work no longer). As the mother of sons, who I assumed—wrongly, I later learned—would be free of cancer problems (only 1 percent of breast cancer occurs in men), I did not then worry too much about passing whatever I carried on my gene-packed forty-six chromosomes (twenty-three from my mother, twenty-three from my father) to the next generations.

A slide flashed on the overhead screen by psychiatrist Mary Jane Massie at a Sloan-Kettering "Genetics and Breast Cancer" seminar changed my thinking. It showed a painting by an American impressionist, Edward Henry Potthast, of three little girls, their curls secured with flouncy satin bows, dancing "Ring around the Rosy" on a beach. The colorful, carefree, happy seaside image startled me. These happy little girls reminded me of my beautiful granddaughters and of the nieces to whom I send valentines each year and whose birthdays and other landmark events I mark as best I can.

"Think of the next generations," I heard Dr. Massie, director of the Barbara White Fishman Center for Psychological Counseling at Sloan-Kettering's Breast Cancer Center, say. "Think of the next generations and consider genetic counseling." I started counting. Ten of my mother's great-grandchildren, ten of my grandmother Linda's great-great-grandchildren, are girls—ranging in age from roughly three to twenty-three. I had been listening, interested but uninvolved, as first the chair, my doctor

Thomas Fahey, and then the intense genetics service chief, Dr.
Kenneth Offit, and breast service chief, Dr. Patrick Borgen, a
genial, caring surgeon, laid out the unpleasant realities: there
are now more than 180,000 new cases a year (1 in every 8 American women) and 40,000 deaths from breast cancer—566 new
cases and 120 deaths each day.

A propensity toward breast cancer (carried in a specific gene)
occurs in only 5 to 10 percent of all the women afflicted by this
most common of female cancers. But, these experts emphasized,
the presence of a BRCA1 or BRCA2 mutation does *not* necessarily mean development of the disease; your genetic constitution
is *not* your destiny; many environmental factors influence it—
what you breathe (smoke included!) and drink, for example, how
you exercise, and the amount of stress in your life may play a
part. So can the care you take to start breast screening early or to
stay away from excess estrogen, be it from oral contraceptives or
hormone replacement therapy.

Still, the breast cancer risk for women who did inherit a
mutated version of the gene from either parent increases over a
lifetime from 12 percent to 60 percent to 80 percent (some say
90 percent). Other depressing discoveries: the risk for breast and
perhaps for ovarian cancer (probably my grandmother's neme-
sis) may be higher among Ashkenazi Jewish women, who are
descendants of northern or non-Sephardic Europeans, than
among women generally. That includes me, my siblings, and our
female descendants. And it can be carried by men like my sons
and nephews as well (leaving them perhaps more vulnerable to
colon, prostate, and even pancreatic cancers).

Dr. Massie, a tall, brisk, empathetic, and, I had always
thought, rather glamorous psychiatrist, described the potential
problems as well as benefits of genetic counseling and genetic
testing. It could cause anxiety, of course, but with professional
counseling this could be avoided. And it could induce worries
that private genetic information about your propensity toward
disease could leak out through computer databases, destroying,
for example, a girl's chances for insurance coverage or even for
suitable employment. This made me sit up and take even more
notice: as someone who once directed a health records confiden-

tiality commission, I am deeply committed to medical privacy.

I was not thinking so much about myself. When I arrived at Sloan-Kettering in the 1970s, I sometimes joke, they looked in my eyes and took out my ovaries (a step designed to induce menopause and thus limit the amount of estrogen in my body). Too late for boobless and ovaryless me to worry about prevention. Now, I learned, if I indeed carried a BRCA1 or BRCA2 mutation, a small chance of my getting something resembling ovarian cancer did exist.

Still, Dr. Massie's image of happy little girls caused me to think primarily about my mother's ten great-granddaughters. If I had genetic counseling, I mused, I could figure out whether I should undergo genetic testing. After all, if the gene definitely lurked in our family, steps could be taken short of drastic prophylactic mastectomy or oophorectomy. My mother's descendants—both women and men—could, for instance, be sure to get early mammograms and other breast, ovarian, colon, and prostate cancer screening; they could stay away from estrogen; they could continue to live healthy lives (with no smoking, of course, veggie-heavy and fat-thin diets, and plenty of exercise).

They might even participate in or make good use of the most up-to-date research of their time—now, for example, that would be in trials testing chemo-preventive drugs like tamoxifen and raloxifene. While no such effort, even drastic surgery, fully guarantees prevention, they maximize the chances that cancer, if it does develop, will be detected at an early enough stage to be successfully treated and that their bodies will be in such good shape that they will tolerate it well.

After the seminar, I discussed my family tree with Tom Fahey, as recommended by the seminar experts for women like me, in "cancer families." He hadn't realized, he said, how many girls there were in my family; indeed, they might be at risk. Then, Dr. Massie and I addressed the anxiety that might be caused if I did carry the suspect gene. She suggested I get the information and send it around to the appropriate family members in sealed envelopes—to be opened or discarded as they wished. This made sense.

I decided to move ahead. The genetic testing some weeks later seemed a piece of cake after some of the procedures I had been through at Sloan-Kettering. In a pleasant, freshly painted room I talked first to Judy Hull, one of the only some one thousand trained genetic counselors in our country. This olive-skinned young woman, a Columbia and Sarah Lawrence graduate, had come to Sloan-Kettering from the University of Washington lab of well-known geneticist Mary Claire King. Careful and deliberate, she radiated an air of competence and calm.

Together, we went over the family tree drawn from information elicited by telephone a few days before—a strange but powerful image in which circles depict women and squares men; black blobs, cancer; and a line through either, death. So I, a circle, have several black blobs but as yet no black line running through me. Later we were joined by the slight but formidable Genetics chief, Dr. Offit, a modern-day medical Sherlock Holmes, earnest and concentrated, pouncing ferretlike on this fact and that as we tried to piece my medical family puzzle together.

The session increased my confidence about the privacy in which my testing results would be kept (their database had never suffered any leakage, said Dr. Offit, knocking wood); all personal identifiers would be removed and coded for research purposes. But our discussion underlined my family's risk. My chances of harboring a BRCA1 or BRCA2 mutation were increased by the facts that I got cancer relatively early (while I was still menstruating), that I had had the disease in both breasts, and that there were multiple cases in my family across the generations.

And the importance of the cause of my grandmother's death—perhaps from ovarian, perhaps metastatic breast cancer—could not be overlooked. Born in 1877, she died in 1936, over sixty years ago. It would be difficult, but they would try to find her records on Sloan-Kettering microfilm.

I signed the consent forms for the genetic testing and was then introduced to Jane Fey, the tall, smiling administrator who coordinates the Metropolitan New York Registry—part of an international National Cancer Institute–funded project. In the cause of research, I consented to be part of this registry collecting anonymous blood samples and epidemiologic data from high-risk families for future studies on breast cancer risk, and I headed with Jane for the laboratory.

An unpleasant surprise: instead of the finger pin prick I expected, the phlebotomist drew seven—count them, seven— vials of blood, two for the genetic testing and five for the research project, a procedure that left my blood-compromised body faint and wobbly and sent a sympathetic Jane scurrying for orange juice and an easy chair. (Had I not participated in the registry, I would have had to part with only two vials.)

Another surprise: to avoid further blood drawing and further questioning, I decided against going into free clinical trials, one at a more convenient medical center, and to follow up privately at Sloan-Kettering. It was expensive ($470 instead of the $270 I had expected) and for the most part not covered by insurance; Caveat Emptor, breast cancer survivors who cannot be worked into appropriate research programs that would pick up the tab. And it would be some time before I got the results.

So we have no solution to my medical mystery as I write, nor will I report it outside the family when I do have it because of the dangers to their privacy such a move might entail. Who knows? Down the pike in the twenty-first century, before my mother's great-grandchildren ever reach my age, the day may come when they and their descendants could have treatments that will repair the mutated genes that tell cancer cells to divide so ruthlessly—and do so without harming healthy cells nearby.

Meanwhile, my hope is that the effort I have put into genetic testing will increase the chances that those I love can at most avoid, and at least alleviate, the pain and trauma of breast—and perhaps other—cancers. And that if they choose to learn the information I uncover, helped by so many, they will meet it head-on, considering it a heartfelt gift they can accept and, if necessary, act on.

9 ✌ *The Media and the Message*
Cancer as Metaphor

October—a lovely time of year in Washington, D.C. In bed, I rested, recovering from my mastectomy operation, as one did twenty-five years ago. I felt pretty good. My recovery had been speedy. The nodes under my arm had proved negative; the doctors told me they felt optimistic about my future.

Then I tuned in to the Nightly News to hear John Chancellor discussing First Lady Betty Ford's recent operation. "Breast cancer," he reported, "is a killer," and he proceeded to prove it with statistics. In 1974 breast cancer was the most common form of death for women between the ages of thirty-one and fifty-five (with the estimated number of new cases more than doubled from 89,000 to over 180,000 in 1998, it is the second major cause, after lung cancer).

Something about the blunt, cool presentation of this information by someone I did not even know started me thinking: even if, as he intoned, the five-year chances for survival after localized breast cancer were about 75 percent (a rate that has now happily soared as high as 97 percent), one of the unlucky 25 percent might just happen to be me. A dark thought. I remembered the words of a J. D. Salinger hero: "It didn't make me feel too gorgeous."

The newsman had turned cancer specialist minus white coat and stethoscope. From him, and from his colleagues in all the media, I learned that 32,500 women (now up to 43,500) would die of the disease in 1974. Worse: the five-year chances for survival declined dramatically if the breast cancer had spread to the axillary (armpit) lymph nodes.

I shut off my television set, blaming Chancellor and company for bringing me this news, without regard for my feelings or sensitivities. This was not quite fair, of course. Common sense and experience told me the messengers should not be blamed for the message. It also told me that message maker and messenger were tied with each other and with me, inextricably, and that both could have presented the message in a more careful, tactful, and empathetic way.

Back then, I do not think anyone gave much thought to how cancer news affected us survivors. On one, minimal end of the scale, when I began chemo, my son Jeremy sent me a clipping from *Newsweek* headlined: "Icy Aid for Cancer Victims." It reported a new technique to spare patients taking chemotherapy the indignity of hair loss. While Adriamycin was being administered, nurses at the University of Arizona fashioned ice packs to cool the scalps of cancer "victims" (few would dare use that word anymore!). This prevented their hair follicles from absorbing the drug, and 70 percent of the patients retained most of their hair.

Since I was on Adriamycin and losing my hair, I rushed to my oncologist, asking for such an ice pack. He nixed the idea. Breast cancer patients can suffer metastases to the scalp; he saw no reason for making the effort I was making and then not having the drugs reach potentially malignant sites for the sake of cosmetics. I thought that over and agreed. I felt disappointed—but nothing lost.

At the other end of the scale a few years later, the *Washington Post* front-paged a sensational headline, "Experimental Drugs: Death in the Search for Cures." Two young investigative reporters had begun a series in which they detailed the gruesome effects of so-called Phase 1, or experimental, anticancer drugs. As the week wore on, I got more and more nervous about the articles because the reporters did not seem to distinguish sufficiently between experimental drugs, which are given only when standard therapies have failed, and routine chemotherapy, with its nuisancelike but bearable (for most people) side effects.

I was right to be nervous. As a New York social worker told me, when she described the negative effect these articles had on her area's survivors, "Cancer patients find articles." People on chemotherapy soon deluged the *Post* with letters telling how the treatment had helped them. Oncologists observed survivors about to begin chemo fearful and dismayed. One of my doctor's patients refused treatment. The gung-ho articles, anxious to make points, right or wrong, about the administration of a small group of drugs to a small group of people, had profoundly troubled a larger group of survivors.

The more things change, the more they remain the same. Certainly they have changed in the decade and a half since that dismaying chemo story appeared. An explosion of information in the world of cancer research has meant more news to report as well as more prospective treatments. More cancer-centered organizations, from government to patient education and advocacy groups to health care professional societies and pharmaceutical companies, vie for attention, sometimes with competing stories. An explosion of information sources, from the classic—though revamped and more user-friendly—newspaper to the Internet, is overeager for solid information about progress in cancer research.

Media people have changed, too; many pay more thoughtful attention to the quality of their reporting than used to be the case. As Victor Cohen, a former science editor and now Visiting Fellow at the Harvard School of Public Health, pointed out during a 1998 communications conference at Cold Spring Harbor, New York, there is today far more good science and medical reporting than there used to be.

But things remain the same, too. There is still plenty that is bad or mediocre (more on the TV news than in print, but often enough in print), which, according to Vic, comes as the result of three "sins" or problems with the work of editors, news directors, and reporters when they:

1. Tend to "believe" what they hear, *if* it's a good story. They fail far too often to apply some of the very simple rules of science and

statistics that can help us separate the truth from trash. Many overlook the power of large numbers to confer believability, and conversely the questionability of stories based on anecdotes or studies of small numbers of people—or animals. (I agree that "a lot of animal stories ain't going to pan out in men and women"; I think of the many well-meaning presenters I have heard at survivor meetings—particularly those speaking of alternative medicine studies—who talk of stressed mice as though they were blood brothers dealing with the same rotten job or nagging marital experiences that stress human beings.)

2. "Hype" or go overboard to get attention for a questionable medical story, whether it promises "New Hope" or "No Hope"—with the former generally the rule. In the process, they may omit or fail to stress the fact that "New Hope" nostrums do not work for everyone, do not always keep working, and are so expensive that many patients cannot use them. (Such stories appeal particularly to survivors already living with disease, and some fine reporters I know are particularly aware of this fact. For example, Susan Okie, a medical doctor who is Vic's former *Post* colleague, now goes to very few scientific meetings at which incremental—step-by-step and often premature—research results are presented, preferring to wait for peer-reviewed articles from the journals she respects most, notably the *New England Journal of Medicine, Annals of Internal Medicine,* and *Lancet.* For instance, she passed on what she considered a marginal though hyped-up report presented at a professional meeting on the efficacy of bone marrow transplant [BMT] for ovarian cancer, telling the publicist who pitched it to her she would wait for the publication of more conclusive proof of the effect of BMT on this nasty disease.)

3. Fail to put news in context. In such cases, they write stories that are incomplete when it comes to what viewers or readers would want to know, especially for intelligent decision making. (All right, will antioxidants keep me from getting a recurrence of my cancer or won't they?) Or they fail to report a whole picture. (The National Coalition for Cancer Survivorship office told me of excited callers asking how to get a new "vaccine" to ward off melanoma reported on TV news; not all but some reports based on a scientific journal

article did not explain clearly enough that this is a treatment, not a preventive vaccine, that has long been tried in patients.)

Of course, responsibility for reporting well on cancer and all health news does not fall only on the shoulders of journalists. It falls also on those of scientist-researchers and medical editors who publish their findings in journals of varying quality (who also employ people to market their wares for public consumption). Such editors do not always remember that their audience now includes not only hundreds of medical print and TV newspeople but physicians who treat patients and also the ultimate users, including me and my fellow survivors, whose question is: "What does this mean to me—and/or those I care about?"

What indeed? The truth is that the changing dynamic between patient and doctor has created survivors and cancer families and friends hungry for reliable information about cancer—information that can be used to ask questions and participate in medical decision making. It cannot be said often enough: We survivors no longer feel content in the role of passive *patients.* We want to know now—ASAP—not only about possible or even probable cures but also how to prevent recurrence in ourselves and occurrence in our families, and we want to achieve an acceptable quality of life while we remain on board to live it. This is a tall order.

And because it is so tall and our needs so complex, we tend to look on sources of information a bit differently than the general public. According to a National Health Council survey released at the end of 1997, most Americans (40 percent) say that television is their top health news source, surpassing doctors, who are the top source for 36 percent (those with increasing levels of education pointing to more reliance on written forms of news in magazines, newspapers, and journals). In contrast, 45 percent of the people with chronic health conditions, including cancer, relied first on health care providers; next, if that source failed or dried up or simply needed confirmation, on print media; and third, on television.

This survey surprised me, and many savvy people I know, by reporting that only a tiny percentage of Americans (2 percent) turn to the Internet as their primary source of information. This probably is changing and will change more as this new communications technology develops effective mechanisms for self-policing and for quality control over health news postings. It will change, too, as more and more people access the Internet, cruising it with an experienced eye for quality information—some of it from major university and research centers—to discuss with their medical caretakers. Of course, even a tiny percentage of our vast population means several million people, so that each significant cancer story, or nonstory, results in many thousands of hits on cancer-related Web sites.

The small survey percentages notwithstanding, anecdotal evidence of Internet power among cancer survivors is strong. One survivor in a Canadian medical center challenges the judgments made by the medical team making grand rounds with an avalanche of information about possible treatments for his cancer. Another reveals in the pages of *Surviving* (reprinted from *Newsweek*) that "when I became physically ill isolated with cancer, my computer brought family and friends to me"; *wired,* he and his wife expanded their horizons and found unimagined support and sources of information. And in a recent issue of the *Washington Post*'s Health section, I read how a Fairfax, Virginia, couple turned with great success to "a new player on the health team," cyberspace, for information on his rare form of lymphoma (MCL), while they pursued more traditional routes. A *Wall Street Journal* headline sums it up: "Medicine: Patients Delve into Databases to Second-Guess Doctors."

Be that as it may, even the most cyber-savvy Internet surfers may get bogged down searching for what the *Journal of the National Cancer Institute* has called "credible and useful Web sites" among the flood of documents on "everything from radical prostatectomy to reflexology, immunotoxins to coffee enemas, gene therapy to walnut juice." The expectation is that in the future, shoddy—even quack—Web sites will atrophy and/or be eliminated (after all, it takes money and sustained effort to keep up a site). If survivors take such unreliable or irrelevant sources at face value, they are likely to be among those (roughly half the general population, according to National Health Council survey results) who consider health news reporting unsatisfactory, or even among those (a whopping 68 percent, according to the same survey) who note that media reports often contradict one another.

Whether surfing the Internet or reading or listening to fast-breaking competitive news reports, the sad truth is that Americans, including some eight million cancer survivors, often do not know what to believe. As we all know, for instance, the confusion about what vitamins might help ward off cancer and its recurrence seems outdone only by the question of how much alcohol one should or can safely imbibe.

Should we have one or two drinks a day to prevent heart attacks (look at the French and their *vin rouge!*) or just wine and beer and no hard booze (though how much you drink seems to be safer than the proof, or what you drink)? But go easy—alcohol is implicated in 3 percent of all cancer deaths, and those who abuse it predispose themselves to certain cancers, including oral and breast tumors. Personally, I have settled on one glass of non-tangy wine a day.

Confusion. This seems to me to be one of two main problems resulting from the way medical science news is presented today. Sometimes, the confusion might mean only the difference between taking an antioxidant vitamin compound as a preventative and taking multivitamins containing vitamins A and D (given to babies in cod liver oil to *make* things grow) or simply vitamin E (a no-no this week).

But more serious issues can stir up a storm, causing the message makers (be they scientists or public policy leaders) to blame the media/messengers and vice versa. The breast cancer screening controversy is a case in point. When this issue surfaced in the press in the late 1970s, I was not particularly aware of it: I had not even had mammography before my first surgery because my surgeon, feeling my breasts so dense that this new tool would not be worth the radiation risks then involved, relied primarily on frequent clinical examinations (CBEs). And I had had few mammograms of my remaining breast.

So I paid little attention when the very first National Institutes of Health (NIH) Consensus Development Conference recommended in 1977 that screening mammography should be available for women over fifty. Women between forty and forty-nine with a personal history of breast cancer or whose mothers or sisters had breast cancer should continue to be screened in an National Cancer Institute–American Cancer Society (NCI-ACS) nonrandomized study called the Breast Cancer Detection Demonstration Project.

The results of this trial, presented in the slow, step-by-step ways of medical science a decade later, implied that younger women would benefit from screening to the same degree as older women. I had by this time lost my remaining breast to a new primary. But, as an active survivor, I had grown more conscious of mammography, knew it now involved fewer risks, and began to follow the evolving story and try to make sense of it. This was no easy job, as any recap of its flip-flop development makes clear. At the 1998 "Breakthrough" conference, journalist Kirsten Boyd Goldberg's presentation helped me to sift through some of the history behind the mammography debate:

> *1987.* A bunch of organizations, including the NCI and the ACS, got together to establish a consensus and produced guidelines recommending annual CBEs with screening mammography every one to two years beginning at age forty; annual CBE and mammography beginning at age fifty; as well as monthly breast self-exams and special surveillance for women with a familial (mother or sister) history of breast cancer.
>
> *1988.* New analysis of a Health Insurance Plan of New York study released a year earlier (which had shown a 30 percent mortality reduction in women over fifty who had had screening mammography, but could not show a benefit for women forty to forty-nine) now showed that of the women who were followed for many years, there were 24 percent fewer breast cancer deaths among women who were screened at forty to forty-nine than in the control group. The cancer organizations now publicized their 1987 guideline widely as a possibly life-saving detection device.

1992. Screening applecart upset. The results of the National
Breast Screening Study, published in the *Canadian Medical Association Journal,* showed that women forty to
forty-nine who received mammograms did no better than
the women who were not screened; in fact, they did worse
than the control group. The ensuing tempest continued,
with pro-screening radiologists who treat patients criti-
cizing the Canadian trial and the medical scientists
involved upholding it.

1993. An NCI-convened workshop issued the "Fletcher
report" (after the panel chair, Suzanne Fletcher of the
American College of Physicians), which reviewed the
data available from many studies and found no reduction
in mortality from breast cancer that could be attributed to
screening for the forty to forty-nine age group, but an
"uncertain, and if present, marginal" reduction in about
ten to twelve years. More information was needed, and
ten-year age groupings were "arbitrary and without biologic justification."

Despite rumblings from Capitol Hill and the NCI's
own National Cancer Advisory Board (NCAB), the NCI
changed its guidelines: women forty to forty-nine should
"discuss with a health professional the advisability of
screening with mammography, taking into account family history and other risk factors," and, like their elders,
should all have annual clinical breast examinations. Dr.
Samuel Broder, NCI director at the time, was quoted (and
misquoted) in the press as saying he would recommend
the controversial annual mammograms to an individual
but not to the public "because I don't have the facts."

1996. New data from updated Swedish studies demonstrated
more conclusively a mortality reduction for women forty
to forty-nine. The NCI planned another Consensus
Conference.

1997. Amid a whirlwind of controversy on Capitol Hill and
elsewhere, spurring accusations of caving in to political
pressures, the NIH (not NCI) appointed the panel and held
the Consensus Conference. Its final statement upheld the

each-woman-should-decide-for-herself view; the new
NCI director Dr. Richard Klausner was quoted in the *New
York Times* as being "shocked" by its conclusions.

Determined that younger women should be screened,
members of Congress weighed in with sharp words; a
"Sense of the Senate" resolution urged the NCAB to consider recommending screening for women forty to forty-
nine or direct them to consider guidelines from others.
The ACS came up with its own statement including
younger women. So did the NCAB, whose statement
stressed the consult-with-your doctor approach—a compromise of sorts.

Whew! At the Cold Spring Harbor conference, Dr. Barbara
Rimer (who served on the Fletcher panel, chaired the NCAB, and
currently serves as the NCI's director of Cancer Control and
Prevention) and editor Kirsten Boyd Goldberg squared off: Who
was primarily responsible for this puzzlement—media/messen-
gers or policy/message makers?

Goldberg faulted the latter, though she had a certain amount
of empathy for their dilemmas. Noting that the institute had
not abandoned its recommendation that women age forty to
forty-nine have mammography screening, she pointed out that
the major change at the NCI in 1993 was that it altered the way
in which it presented this information and few members of the
press, including herself, were aware of this decision at the
time. This was because NCI officials alluded to it only subtly
in the NIH's Physician's Data Query (PDQ)—obscure even to
some oncologists—when PDQ stopped referring to screening
guidelines and instead began issuing "summary of evidence"
statements.

What this meant, the newsletter editor explained, was that
rather than accepting trial evidence of "inferential benefit" that
simply happens to show a benefit that is not statistically significant (on which its original women-in-their-forties guideline
was based), the NCI would accept only a "statistically significant benefit." If the agency had been more forthright, she felt
the ensuing process of developing a statement on screening

mammography would not have been so confused and conten-
tious and could have centered on evidence-based medicine.

Instead, the public perception of confusion and diminishing
hope for effective breast cancer screening intensified, and the
final official decision-making process became a "communications disaster." Though she stressed that medicine is changing
and standards are higher than they were twenty years ago, Goldberg observed that the situation worsened as more and more
diverse policy makers got into the act, whether they were
nonexpert panelists or elected officials. And it hit rock bottom
during dialogues like this that took place at one of four separate hearings held before the Senate Labor Appropriations
Subcommittee:

> *Chairman Arlen Specter (R-Pa.):* Dr. Klausner, either I hear you
> saying for the third time that they're wrong or hear you say-
> ing something, candidly, which is unintelligible. The women
> of America in the age category of 40 to 49 need to know in
> unequivocal terms whether a mammogram would be helpful
> to them in detecting breast cancer. Yes or No?
>
> *Dr. Richard Klausner (NCI director):* And, as I said, I hope I have
> been trying to be very clear, and that is that the evidence is,
> as far as I can read . . . that there is a statistically significant
> benefit in terms of reduction of mortality over long periods
> of time from initiating screening at some time in your for-
> ties. I think I have been very clear with that. And as I said, I
> disagree with that aspect of the report of the panel.
>
> *Specter:* I take that as a yes.

Goldberg concluded that though the NCI had not been forthright about its intentions and had not communicated well, this
level of political pressure was uncalled for and "a blatant attack
on science." What's more, scientists and science writers did
little to call politicians on it.

Speaking for the message makers, Dr. Rimer admitted to
being stunned when, after the release of the 1993 Fletcher report,
a popular conclusion gleaned from reporters with varying points
of view was that panelists had capitulated to health care reform
political pressure in limiting its screening recommendation (and

so public health expenditures). Later, when the NCAB panel she chaired issued its statement for women in their forties, politics and conflict, particularly on Capitol Hill, again seemed to her to make a more interesting story than the complexity of science (whose results often do not seem to translate well into social policy).

This is true, Dr. Rimer explained in a talk titled "Older and Wiser," because data are messy, policy setting is difficult, and, very often, how one interprets the data depends on where one sits (the epidemiologist/scientists use a public health yardstick; the primarily radiologist/physicians, an individual patient benefit yardstick). To improve reporting, she felt the press should apply the rules of evidence in explaining the complexity of issues—whether the data are plausible, for instance, the sample is of sufficient size, and the design adequate. And though later analysis showed, in some cases at least, that the NCAB panel deliberations coverage wasn't as one sided as she had perceived at the time, she still felt the media's challenge is to simplify without being simplistic: "The price we all pay for sound bites may be obfuscation."

True indeed. When, in the late 1990s, my daughter-in-law Debbie asked me what breast cancer screening the authorities recommended for younger women, I had to tell her I was not absolutely sure (and I don't think the rest of the public was either). I thought that the final compromise guidelines recommended some sort of informed decision making, in which she and her doctor would weigh risks and potential benefits of mammography screening and decide on a prudent course of action.

Back into the Arms of the Media. A second survivorship problem grows out of this confusion. When the only advice the scientist/experts can give the public in the midst of scientific uncertainty is "consult your doctor and then do what you think best," you're conveying what might have been fair in the old days. Then, that doctor had an hour or at least half an hour to spend with you, walking you through your options, with their attendant risks and benefits.

Now, the doctor, whether practicing in a managed care or fee-for-service setting, operates in a ten- to fifteen-minute time frame. Since it is next to impossible to have any sort of prolonged, informed, and informing dialogue in that time, the bulk of the decision-making burden can, and often does, shift back to you, the patient. You can, of course, shop for second and third opinions—if you have the time and wherewithal and your health care system allows you to do so. And/or you can be thrown back into the arms of the media—be it print, audiovisual, or Internet—that told you to consult your doctor in the first place.

No wonder that cancer organizations often rely on individual survivor stories, rather than scientific reports, to get their messages across. Though scientists and ace science writers may frown on the use of anecdotes and personal accounts, a good section of the public identifies with and responds to them, particularly when they involve widely known VIPs. Of course, this practice is not risk-free: celebrity images may change, or their popularity may wane or wax in a way that overpowers a message; there may even be a certain amount of resentment against gorgeous Hollywood types speaking authoritatively about fields they know little about.

Still, credible VIPs can help greatly in conveying a message. This might be a message of prevention and hope (e.g., a lung-cancer-stricken Yul Brynner urging people not to smoke as he, alas, had; or Candace Bergen's prime-time portrayal of a feisty Murphy Brown dealing with breast cancer in an episode punctuated by a set of consciousness-raising infomercials about early detection—bought by the Ford Motor Company for the Susan G. Komen Breast Cancer Foundation. The episode elicited almost two thousand telephone calls in just three days). Or it might be a message of survivorship (Betty Ford straightforwardly lifting hearts as she opened the breast cancer closet; General Norman Schwarzkopf urging others to march with him to conquer cancer and its consequences—including the aloneness he felt before he found other men with whom he could share prostate cancer information and experiences).

Survivorship messages can be presented particularly effectively when highly respected private persons step forward to tell public cancer tales. Introducing Supreme Court Justice Sandra Day O'Connor to an audience of survivors (and through the marvel of cable television, live and nationwide), I remembered that, when I had once worked happily for then Senator and later Vice President Hubert Humphrey, Muriel Humphrey used to say that she felt she held a "magic wand" as a result of their public position—a magic wand that she could use to benefit others.

Nothing was so gratifying to us involved in survivorship work, I continued, as the emergence of an eminent public servant like Justice O'Connor or former senator Paul Tsongas before her, who was willing to wave her or his magic wand for us. Her presence at our annual assembly made others "more aware that there is a life after cancer, and that it can be enormously productive, and even fun." And I added it made us feel that, though we may not be Supreme Court justices or serious presidential candidates such as lymphoma survivor Tsongas (and later prostate cancer survivor Senator Bob Dole), if we worked hard and had some smarts, we, too, might be heard, whether in our doctors' offices or in public corridors of power.

Giving that introduction, I did not dream that Sandra Day O'Connor's ensuing candid account of her breast cancer experiences (see chapter 2) would move survivors nationwide, making them feel that if a brilliant Supreme Court justice could feel the same anxiety, the same stress, weariness, and confusion they knew so well, they could not be as inadequate—as *dumb*—as they had thought. What's more, O'Connor's presence and its ripple effects through wide media coverage improved not only our image of ourselves but also the public's perception of survivorship.

No wonder, then, that embryonic organizations like the Ovarian Cancer National Alliance (OCNA) look for prominent role models during a start-up phase. OCNA, game for a cutesy slogan ("Ovar'coming Together"—which appears quickly during an Internet search), could speak of a few well-known women (Connecticut congresswoman Rosa DeLauro, twenty-four-year survivor and former Miss America Bess Myerson, and *Harper's Bazaar* editor in chief Liz Tilberis) willing to follow the late actor-comedian Gilda Radner in speaking openly and personally about the disease. *Ms.* magazine speculated (in April 1998) that the reluctance of others to follow suit may be explained by a hesitance to be seen as a doomed victim of what is perceived to be an inevitably fatal disease.

Susan Sontag, in her classic *Illness as Metaphor,* pioneered in calling attention to this false perception. In addition to the pain and loss of the disease itself, survivors have traditionally had to shoulder another burden: a stigmatized image tarnished by the dishonor, the shame, of having contracted a disreputable, most possibly fatal, evil. Once, as Sontag explained, it was the more romantic passive disease tuberculosis; now—perhaps to a lesser degree than twenty years ago—it is still cancer, which seems to many to secretly and ruthlessly invade and corrode people and institutions.

Though cancer has been known to human beings for a long, long time (ancient Egyptian writings refer to tumors and primitive means of treatment—by knife), they have never come to regard it as ordinary. Thousands of years have only mystified the disease process and those afflicted with it. Cancer, a word that comes from the Greek *karkinos* and the Latin *cancer* (both meaning "crab"), has through the ages been associated with a sense of dread and evil. It is obscene in the original sense of the word: ill omened, abominable, repugnant to the senses.

Despite all the work we survivors have done to show others that we can live quite satisfactory lives, a taboo often surrounds us, as it once surrounded people with tuberculosis. Nothing of that taboo is attached to people with cardiac disease, an illness implying merely weakness, trouble, mechanical failure. In his beautiful book *At the Will of the Body,* Canadian survivor Arthur Frank describes the differences in how others perceived him when he suffered a heart attack and when he developed testicular cancer. After the heart attack, he reports, they said, "You've really bounced back," a phrase not repeated after his cancer. This was true, thought this medical sociologist, because in most cases we do not sink into an experience, we only hit the surface, while with cancer, he was going "to have to sink all the way through to discover a life on the other side."

For cancer is not just a disease. In English, and other lan-
guages, the word has been applied figuratively to social, political, and other human enterprises. "Sloth is a Cancer, eating up
that Time, Princes should cultivate for Things sublime," wrote
Edmund Ken in 1711, Susan Sontag reports. She cites many
other examples of the use of the word *cancer* to describe corro-
sion of what was considered the social good: John Adams wrote
in his diary in 1772 that "Venality, Servility and Prostitution
spread like a cancer." Trotsky called Stalinism a cancer that
must be burned out with a hot iron. Somewhat differently, D. H.
Lawrence called masturbation "the deepest and most dangerous
cancer of our civilization." And we all know how John Dean
explained Watergate to Richard Nixon: "We have a cancer
within—close to the Presidency—that's growing."

So every survivor carries around the language of cancer as a
synonym, not only for death, but for demoralization and devas-
tation. To rectify the conception of the disease, argues Sontag,
would make it less something to hide; but like tuberculosis, it
will remain so until its etiology becomes clear and its treatment
effective. Acquiring this understanding, unfortunately, is turning into a long process.

Arguably, this has begun, with medical advances and with the
emergence of long-term survivors into full public view. We now
see not the end but the clear ebb of a startling consequence of
stigma—the belief that we all must be on guard against cancer,
since it might be *contagious.* Certainly we no longer hear of the
public quarantine of cancer patients. And we hear less of more
personal hang-ups—of house hunters turned off by the news that
the previous owner of a desirable residence had cancer, or of
couples whose sex life wanes after one develops cancer; the pair
may know better intellectually, but, as one wife put it, though
she knew "logically" that she could not contract cancer "that
way," once in bed something else took over and she "couldn't do
it."

People who occupy public positions, even in settings of supposed acceptance and worth, have had special trouble confronting the unhappy reputation of cancer and the rejecting
behavior it can evoke. I can remember Israel's Golda Meir keep-

ing the knowledge of her disease secret for more than a decade before she died in 1978, rather than risk sharing it with the public. In the dark of the night, she would go for her radiation treatments, preferring this subterfuge to endangering her political fortunes and those of her government.

In our country, which had achieved a more open use of the word *cancer,* the proponent of the politics of joy who died in the same year did not have to hide his cancer. To the contrary, Hubert Humphrey was able to be open and truthful about his disease, whether setting an example on TV or striding about hospital corridors in his bathrobe, encouraging fellow patients and delighting the staff. He accepted from his doctors information about the progress of his bladder disease beyond the perimeter of surgery. Still, this same information anguished both Humphrey and his family when it appeared on television and in print news stories, bombarding him with cold, negative statistics; he felt like a horse in the Belmont stakes.

Less than two decades later, public understanding of cancer (and the chances for survival) had increased enough that VIPs like Senators Dole and Tsongas—though they certainly did not advertise the fact of their cancer at campaign time—dared toss their hats into the presidential ring. Yet Justice O'Connor confessed that the "worst" for her had been her public visibility through constant media coverage. She said that the press kept asking, "How does she look? When is she going to step down and give the President another vacancy on the Court? She looks pale to me, I don't give her six months. This was awful."

More than that, O'Connor said "there were people in the press box with telescopes looking at me in the courtroom to see just what my condition was. I didn't like that. Press would call my office and say they'd heard all these dire rumors and I better tell them exactly what was what or they were going to publish them all. It was really difficult."

More ordinary women and men do not have to worry about people in the press box with telescopes. But we survivors do have to worry about a certain amount of *scapegoatism* simply because we have cancer. Often we are made to feel we are at fault, simply because of our disease.

The nurse who accosted me in my hospital room, wanting to know why my breast cancer had metastasized (see chapter 2), serves as a dramatic example. Why hadn't I talked to the doctor about avoiding spread? Why hadn't I gone in for regular check-ups? She made me so uncomfortable that I should not have been surprised, a few years later, at the enthusiastic survivor response to my Cancer Survivors' Bill of Rights stipulation that in their personal lives, survivors have the right not only to be free of the stigma of cancer as a "dread disease" but also "to be free of blame for having gotten the disease and having survived it."

The sort of crude tactlessness this nurse displayed is grounded in absolute faith in the survivor's ability to control her own medical destiny, the false notion that if only you had obeyed the medical rules, you would be in the clear. Beyond this there are more subtle attitudes that inflict guilt on patients. There is the perhaps unconscious feeling that we get what we deserve in this world and that there must be some justice in one's fate. Of course, if a survivor has brought the disease on him- or herself, others protect themselves from vulnerability to it and, if they wish, absolve themselves from responsibility for helping.

We survivors recognize these uncomfortable attitudes particularly when they are reflected in media stories. If only we had lived right! If only we had jogged, or eaten in a nutrition-wise fashion, or enjoyed more emotional fulfillment—loving more successfully, loving *ourselves* more and developing a stronger will to resist disease!

There is no medical quarrel, of course, with the don't smoke and drink-in-moderation advice. But some doctors, including the late distinguished doctor-poet Lewis Thomas, have pointed out that it's the healthy people who are apt to be out there jogging. What's more, admonitions about healthy living may not apply in individual cases, in which a host of factors, including heredity and environment, play significant parts.

But it is the compelling idea that through positive feelings like love and hope survivors can influence the course of their disease, popularized particularly in the 1980s by the former Yale surgeon and cancer guru Dr. Bernie Siegel, that seems to me to have the potential for special mischief. For when hanging-in patients polish their self-image and in other ways follow Bernie-like suggestions (even making drastic lifestyle changes, like divorcing spouses) and do not feel better—when their disease, alas, may progress despite their efforts to change—they may feel themselves not only severely punished but also at fault.

When I spoke out about such issues in a *Washington Post* review of Siegel's book *Peace, Love, and Healing,* I received one of my most treasured fan letters, from the late Dr. Karl Menninger, saying he had been enthusiastic about Siegel's earlier work that emphasized the humanity of patients who need hope and encouragement, not just diagnosis, pills, and manipulations. But, after reading the proofs of this second book, he had urged—because of the sort of questions I had raised—that it not be published.

To no avail. The cancer self-help message that this former surgeon and others touted seeped out into our culture through the media, adding a modern get-your-act-together-or-else aspect to the already ugly image of the disease and leaving many pained casualties. One woman I met reported sitting on the toilet all day after a second cancerous obstruction was diagnosed, crying as she read an article, in a magazine she had picked up in the supermarket, about people who had gotten the upper hand over their cancers. Why couldn't she do that?

Better to insist that our disease is just that, a disease for which the cause or causes are still, unfortunately, murky—a phenomenon of nature still not completely understood. Better to know that the 1990s, with their explosion of knowledge, have cleared the way for exciting progress in the next century by establishing as ludicrous the notion that we survivors are—somehow—absolutely responsible and to blame for our cancer. That is the healthiest way of hanging in.

And as we will see, we need to hang in healthy to be fit to combat cancer's evil image—what at least one survivor calls "cancerphobia."

10 ✤ *Work*
The Passion of Labor

When her Long Island lawyer-boss fired legal secretary Jane Karuschkat, he fired the wrong person—though he did not know it at the time. Jane, a breast cancer survivor who missed less than a week of work (a combination of sick leave and vacation days) after her mastectomy, fought back. She lost her job. But she won the suit she filed against the lawyer to the tune of $70,000. And, despite a metastasis to her hip, a prophylactic second mastectomy, and repeated bouts with lymphedema (swelling in the arms), she gained a serene and accomplished quality of life and a new double career as an artist and advocate for the rights of cancer survivors in the workplace.

A perky forty-one-year-old in the fall of 1992, Jane enjoyed her job and felt appreciated and productive at the busy five-lawyer office as she was awarded her annual Christmas bonus. Her co-workers supported and encouraged her when she developed cancer and underwent first a lumpectomy, then a mastectomy, and scheduled her semimonthly chemotherapy (on Fridays after work so she would have her off-duty weekends to recover). She relied on her job, not only for the paycheck, which helped at home while her husband, Glenn, established a new business, but for familiar routine tasks that gave her a feeling of stability as her cancer diagnosis turned her world "upside down, chaotic and topsy-turvy." She felt better knowing she held a steady job.

She had the mastectomy on a Friday, rearranged the furniture in her hospital room on Saturday, and came home from the hospital on Sunday. When she called her law firm's office manager, she got the first sign that she was going to be given a hard time. She was told she could not return as planned on Tuesday; she needed a note from her doctor giving her permission to work (when she went to the doctor's office to pick it up, he asked if her boss thought she was still in kindergarten). Next thing she knew, a special messenger arrived carrying disability forms. Rather than sign them, she returned to work the next day. Looking back, she remembers people acting extra "nice" to her—perhaps too nice. When she asked if she could help with this chore or that, they would not let her. Still, she hoped things would soon return to normal.

Jane felt rotten after her first chemotherapy treatment in January, so she took another of her accumulated sick leave days, stayed home on Monday, and went back to work on Tuesday. On Friday, her boss called her into the office library. "This is going to be as hard for me as it is for you," he began. He could not, he continued, afford to keep her any longer. She smelled what she came to call "cancerphobia"; she felt he really meant "You're going to be sick all the time and I don't want to deal with it. Out!" No one else had been fired, even among those with less seniority, and she had had no indications that her work was not satisfactory. Back at her desk, she cleaned out her drawers and told one of the other lawyers who asked her to take dictation that she did not work there any more. Then she called her husband to pick her up. She had been thrown out in the cold, with a week's severance pay (she had asked for two).

She knew one thing: she did not want to sit around. She wanted—she needed—to do something about what had happened to her. As a legal eagle, she had heard about the Americans with Disabilities Act (ADA) enacted by the Congress in 1990, which had taken effect the previous year; she knew that it protected "disabled persons" (including cancer survivors) qualified for a job and able to perform its "essential functions" and that employers must provide them with "reasonable accommodations." She reasoned that other people must have been discriminated against as she had been. Putting a network out, she continued to research her case and started looking for a lawyer

involved in health and employment issues. She considers herself
lucky to have found one in a ball of fire named L. Susan Slavin.

The legal process seldom seems quick or easy. The ADA had
set the stage and changed the atmosphere. But it did not apply to
her case because her company employed fewer than fifteen
people. So Slavin filed a complaint with the New York State
Division of Human Rights. She asked the unprecedented: that
the agency rule in favor of a breast cancer survivor in a discrimination case and that a judge require New York State to extend its
disability law to include the new federal ADA standards man-
dating "reasonable accommodations" for people with disabilities. Jane's former law firm fought the complaint.

After some tough moments, in which Jane had to sit in a hearing room and listen to former colleagues testify against her
(hard, even though she knew they needed to keep their jobs), she
won. She savored the verdict, not so much for its $20,000 award
for lost wages and $50,000 for "mental anguish," but for the
knowledge that her case is now cited in courtrooms throughout
the country, as cancer survivors fight discrimination. It is helping empower people, showing them they should not sit back and
simply take it.

Jane's reputation as a dynamite person preceded her. I found
her to be that and more: a special gutsy woman, with a warm and
loving but not sappy approach to her disease and its aftermath. A
talented artist, she took lessons to become a professional, and
the depth of her feeling for the wonders of the world around her
shows in her paintings, particularly in her landscapes, which
have begun to be exhibited. And she continued to sing at wed-
dings, another vocation she had trained for at several schools,
including the Mannes College of Music. She tries to ice skate
regularly—she loves the cold and the flying feeling she experiences on the ice. Since her case received wide publicity, she has
many invitations to speak and counsel other survivors; she
responds as best she can.

Though not without pain, her life has expanded, and she is
grateful for that and for the fact that she is doing something for
society, however modest, in fighting "cancerphobia" in the
workplace. She considers herself a spiritual person and prays a

good deal to her own vision of force, of energy, of God. She asks that the love, the peace, the serenity she feels continue, that her fears of death be taken away.

Before we hang up, she gives me, as she had when we first met, a telephone hug. A double hug.

Ours is a work-oriented culture; our adult lives center about our jobs. Work is rooted deeply in our society. It establishes our sense of worth, our identity.

Work, as Studs Terkel put it, is about a search "for daily meaning as well as daily bread, for recognition as well as cash, for astonishment rather than torpor; in short, for a sort of life rather than a Monday through Friday sort of dying." In the United States especially, we feel we should earn by our labor for ourselves and our dependents—and this is increasingly true for women as well as men. Our ethic suspects idleness; we say people are "poor but honest"; we suspect "welfare fraud." We tend to measure personal adequacy by the economic independence gained from work. Like Freud, we consider *Lieben und Arbeiten* ("love and work") the two great moving impulses.

In this setting, the cancer survivor can be severely handicapped. "I received a death sentence twice," confided Jon, a forty-two-year-old bookkeeper with a colostomy, "once when my doctor told me I have cancer, then when my boss asked me to quit because the cancer would upset my fellow workers. Except for my wife, that job was my whole world." Jon was one of 277 patients interviewed by Frances Lomas Feldman, a professor of social work, and her researchers for a three-volume study of work-able cancer patients in California. Conducted under the auspices of the state's American Cancer Society Division, this classic study was the first major assessment of work and cancer when it was published in the mid-1970s.

The in-depth Feldman studies of clinically cured cancer survivors—white-collar workers, blue-collar workers, and young people with a "likelihood of prime employability" because of age, education, and ability—brought us some disturbing news from the workplace. Most of the men and women studied were working full- or part-time or were in school. But a good portion of them were unable to find the work they wanted or had had job applications turned down because of their history of cancer.

What's more, job hunting generally required a much greater effort than before the diagnosis. Forty-five percent of the younger workers blamed cancer for their failure to obtain jobs, and nearly three-fourths of these claimed they were told that this was the reason; 23 percent of the blue-collar men and women had either left their precancer employer or been rejected for at least one other job because of their cancer histories. Clues as to why this was so abounded: one person, for instance, was asked to use a pencil rather than a pen in a public employment office; pencils can be discarded more easily!

Yet the cancer survivors' experience in the workplace was not entirely gloomy. Survivors in all three of the studies had positive experiences, which at times outweighed the negative, when they looked for jobs and, later, when they went back to work or school. Some talked about co-workers who were "marvelous," about helpful supervisors and friends who pitched in to help them with strenuous tasks. As a breast cancer survivor put it, "As time went on, I didn't feel that I was so different from other women." Added an ironworker, "I'm feeling desperate when I'm not working. I can't lean over and die at my age [forty-four]. So I've had two bouts! I'll be back at my job soon; they're holding it for me."

I'm feeling desperate when I'm not working. Survivors of all races and ethnic groups in the Feldman studies tried to demonstrate to themselves and others that they were still useful, able to take care of themselves and retain mastery over their lives in spite of cancer. Though some erred in sending out signals that they were unsure they could keep to a job schedule or do a certain job (like a man with a colostomy who brought up his toileting needs several times during an interview and was not hired), most insisted they could carry their own weight and did. They worked harder, faster, better than other people. They performed stressful tasks and were not poor risks. They were rarely absent.

As we will see, this holds true today, with one study showing that typical survivors concur that their job helped them maintain their emotional stability and on average reported missing fewer than five days of work per month during treatment.

I never thought I had experienced workplace discrimination due to my cancer. At the time of my first mastectomy almost a quarter century ago, I was working as an assistant editor for the *Chronicle of Higher Education,* covering health-related topics in anticipation of the newsmagazine's starting a similar health education news magazine. I enjoyed the job. And rifling through old files the other day, I concluded that my bosses could not have been dissatisfied with my work from the number of bylined front-page stories they published—ranging from in-depth analyses of nursing and social work education to reports on science Ph.D.'s studying to be medical doctors (datelined Miami) and courses in sexuality (datelined Detroit).

Indeed, they sent me flowers and kind words when I went into the hospital for surgery. Like most of my fellow survivors, I looked forward to getting out of a recuperative mode, out of the house, back to the stimulation of useful work and friendly colleagues, returning to the job. But when I did so, I was called into the managing editor's office and given the ax.

Perhaps because it was done politely, perhaps because my medical bills were covered by my workplace insurance, perhaps because, like many other survivors of that day, I bought—at least partially—into the managing editor's excuse (I had been hired with an eye to working on a health journal, which they never did get out, and any health education news could be covered by an able, healthwise colleague). In those pre-ADA days, I simply cleaned out my desk and went home without an argument and without even admitting what had happened to me. But I was hurt and worried; nothing similar had ever happened to me before.

Or since. In fact, the jobs I lucked into in the seventies and eighties helped me push the *Chronicle* experience into a shady corner of my mind. For several years, while I was executive director of a small national nonprofit organization, my health professional board of directors extended themselves to accommodate my subsequent hospitalizations and my half-time schedule (true, they got a good bargain: they paid me half-time, and I usually worked three-quarters time, at least).

Later, when Liz Carpenter, whom I had known as a Washington journalist and White House press secretary, called to ask me to take a speech-writing job at the Department of Education, I hesitated, knowing her to be the kind of person who goes at seventy-five thousand miles an hour and has little sympathy for those who drop by the wayside.

"But Liz," I said, "I've been sick." (I had—with bone metastases and subsequent radiation and chemotherapy treatments.)

"That's all right," she answered. "You're better now."

Jimmy Carter's secretary of education, the remarkable Shirley Hufstedler, was a model employer, too, solicitous but not overly so. On a trip to Barnard College, where she delivered the commencement address, she told me she wanted me to do just what I felt like doing, and no more. Such a statement doesn't always come with the territory, even in a large organization like a federal government agency.

But that old experience simmering in a corner of my mind had sent my antennae up. I saw news stories I had not seen before. I read, for example, about a police captain his colleagues dubbed "Captain Chemo." When he found a dead rat in his car and, later, a pile of garbage in his parking space, he did not tell his superiors, thinking that somehow he was at fault for switching his men at a southern Maryland police station from a four- to a five-day work schedule. But when he began to receive threatening phone calls at home, and when his wife got a midnight call in which a man taunted her about her husband's cancer and chemotherapy, he did report the harassment.

I read another Maryland story about Greg Walters, who tried to enlist in the marines. Despite help from his parents, his senator, and the doctors who had treated him for a rare form of lymphoma, he did not make it. Way back then, the U.S. Marine Corps turned him down because he had not been "symptom free" for five years.

Listening to the scholarly Frances Feldman speak at a meeting about her landmark research, I reasoned that if her findings were true in California, the likelihood was that cancer discrimination took place to an even greater degree in other states with no such legislation. After all, California was a state with heightened sensitivity to the issue, a state that since 1976, shortly before her first volume was published, had had a law that specifically forbade employment discrimination against people with "any health impairment related to or associated with cancer."

Yet I still thought such discrimination happened to others, somewhere else. Perhaps this was because I knew that most employers treated survivors fairly and legally—as I had usually been treated. Susan Scherr, a survivor of both breast and uterine cancer, was one such. Susan, who has since held several high positions in the National Coalition for Cancer Survivorship (NCCS), had worked for bosses who were thoroughly supportive through both her cancer episodes—the first, in the 1970s, when she told only her supervisor at her savings and loan trade association job about the reason for her absence from work; the second, a decade later, when everyone in her national personnel placement company "knew" after she fainted in the office and had to be taken to the hospital by rescue squad. Similarly, my own son Jonathan was treated with genuine understanding by his fellow academics in the Mathematics Department at Georgia Tech—told he could take whatever time off he needed and make any working arrangements he wanted during and after treatment for Hodgkin's disease.

My point of view changed in the late 1980s, when I started to work with other cancer survivors among the NCCS leadership—particularly with fellow board member Barbara Hoffman. This slight young attorney, a soft-spoken Hodgkin's disease survivor with long brown hair, was easy to underestimate. But it did not take me long to discover that, though short in stature, she was tall in energy and determination; underneath her Savannah-bred demeanor lurked an acute Princeton-trained mind and tough understanding of the developing field of disabilities law.

At NCCS annual assemblies, and in the pages of the organization's newsletter, the *Networker*, which I founded and edited for five years, Barbara focused our attention on the increasing number of survivors who were encountering a strange phenomenon: modern medicine had enabled them to beat back their cancers (some, particularly among the young people, were considered "cured") and return to the workplace, but modern society had not truly accepted them there. Indeed, studies have suggested that about a quarter of all survivors were encountering workplace discrimination.

Some were fighting back successfully, though they were protected only in a limited way (chiefly by the Federal Rehabilitation Act, which covered only public employees, as well as various state human rights laws). In 1988, for example, a Texas lymphoma survivor named Walter Ray Ritchie won a federal court lawsuit against the city of Houston, which denied him a firefighter's job because of his cancer history. This landmark case marked a victory for survivors who worked for public employers or those receiving federal funds.

Another public employee's case had a different outcome. New York lawyer Timothy Calonita did not really want to be a lawyer; he wanted to be a cop. But when he applied for police officer training and completed all the tests successfully, the Civil Service doctor said, "Whoa—we've got standards here and our standards say we cannot employ anyone who has a history or presence of a malignant tumor." His automatic disqualification changed Tim, who had considered the Hodgkin's disease he'd been successfully treated for as a teenager a "private affair," into an outspoken foe of cancer prejudice.

Tim became one of the team of lawyers Barbara Hoffman was assembling to help survivors with workplace problems. In her *Networker* columns and in testimony before various official bodies, Barbara explained why such action, indeed more formal protection, was needed. In early 1989 she told a Senate Labor and Human Resources Subcommittee that more than a million Americans had experienced some form of job discrimination solely because of their cancer histories. These included:

A paralegal breast cancer survivor fired when she was unable to convince her employer that she had lost her breast, not her brain.

A hotel kitchen employee transferred from his job for fear he
  might "contaminate the food."
A corporate senior executive forced to resign, although he had
  demonstrated that he could perform his job while undergoing cancer treatment.

Such discrimination had taken place, Barbara testified,
despite some telling facts: 80 percent of adult cancer survivors
returned to work successfully after diagnosis. And studies had
shown that they had relatively the same productivity rates as
other workers.

Barbara, meanwhile, ever the persistent attorney (while teaching at several universities and mothering two little girls), counseled cancer survivors in speeches across the country about
furthering their chances in applying for jobs and holding on to
them. Survivors packed her workshops at NCCS assemblies
every year, seeking advice and practical tips. They learned not to
volunteer cancer histories to prospective employers; to remember that in most states questions about your health could only
be asked when they were job related; and not to be too inquisi-
tive about health benefits before getting a firm offer, preferably
in writing.

In Los Angeles in 1988 I heard her outline three "myths"
prevalent in the workplace: that cancer is a death sentence, that
survivors are less productive than other workers, and that cancer is contagious. (One example: the case of a woman who finished treatment for laryngeal cancer and came back to work to
find her desk coated with Lysol.) And in Washington two years
later, she explained, "Even if you don't consider yourself handicapped, if your employer treats you like you are you may have a
case." That really struck home.

Meanwhile, cancer survivor advocates, like Hoffman and
Grace Monaco of the Candlelighters Childhood Cancer Foundation, joined forces with coalitions of other disability rights
activists to work for passage of federal protective disabilities
legislation and to ensure that it would protect cancer survivors.

On July 26, 1990, I stood on the White House lawn—along with
at least a thousand other activists—to watch President George

Bush sign the Americans with Disabilities Act into law. Jeremy
and Debbie, my son and daughter-in-law, called that night from
Boston to complain that they did not see me in the television
coverage of the event. It was no wonder: the sun beat down
fiercely on the crowded ceremony scene, causing many of us to
seek shade under the nearest tree. I neither got close to the center of the action nor accomplished my chief purpose as NCCS's
representative on the scene: to point out to the hordes of media
reporting the story that cancer survivors were a part of it (there
were, ironically, too many more outwardly disabled people
present—a common public relations problem for inwardly disabled cancer survivors).

But nothing dampened my delight in being there or my organization's satisfaction with the event. In fact, the NCCS minutes of a telephone board meeting taking place concurrently
noted that "Natalie was absent because she was at the White
House attending the ceremony marking the signing of the Americans with Disabilities Act!" And, in the next *Networker'* s
"Advocacy Update" column, Barbara Hoffman noted that
although the new law, which would take effect in July 1992,
did not specifically mention cancer survivors, federal courts
and agencies were expected to apply the law to them. ADA, she
explained, would prohibit employment discrimination against a
qualified employee because he or she is disabled, has a history of
a disability, or is regarded as disabled. Specifically, it would:

1. Cover—for a two-year start-up period—private businesses with
   more than twenty-five employees, regardless of whether they
   received federal funding; thereafter it would cover those with
   fifteen or more employees.
2. Prohibit employers from requiring preemployment examinations designed to screen out individuals with a disability, including a cancer history. An employer, under the law, could ask
   medical questions only after someone was offered a job and only
   if the questions were specifically job-related.

We were on our way—or at least further along. And the enact-
ment of the Family and Medical Leave Act (in 1993) added
another layer of protection. The FMLA, for which survivors had

strongly advocated, requires employers of fifty or more employees to provide up to twelve weeks of unpaid, job-protected leave
for family members who need time off to address their own serious illness, to care for a seriously ill child, parent, spouse, or a
healthy newborn or newly adopted child.

Fast-forward to the end of the century. Ask disabilities lawyers
whether the ADA protects cancer survivors from employment
discrimination, and they will answer with an unsatisfactory but
accurate: "Sometimes yes, sometimes no."

The ADA certainly moved us ahead. It not only heightened
survivor expectations for fairer treatment, and thus changed the
workplace atmosphere, but has also had concrete results. Cancer survivors have filed 2 percent of all ADA cases—a number
that represents thousands of cases; many were won or settled
favorably; the law has probably discouraged many other
instances of discrimination.

But, like most laws, ADA cannot be viewed as a quick fix for
working or would-be-working survivors. In a spring 1998 *Networker* "Advocacy Update" column, NCCS counsel Barbara
Hoffman explained why this was so:

To win a case under the ADA, you must show you have a "disability" as defined by the law. This means you must have or have
had a physical or mental impairment that greatly limits (or
used to limit) at least one major life activity, or your employer
believes (rightly or wrongly) you have such an impairment. You
must also show you are able to perform the essential functions
of the job—that you are qualified for that job. And that you were
treated differently *because* of your disability.

The result? A catch-22 for many survivors. If they are too
ill to work, some courts may consider them "unqualified"
under the law. Yet if they are able to work during or after cancer treatment, as new antinausea medicines and other advances have enabled more and more of them to do, courts may
refuse to recognize cancer as a "disability" that is "substantially limiting."

That's what happened to two men who filed cases under ADA
in the 1990s: Paul Hirsch and Michael Boyle. Hirsch's boss

refused his request to work at home two days a week, despite his thirty years of service, and later fired him. A federal court in Illinois threw out his case, on grounds that Hirsch had not shown how his lymphoma, which ultimately killed him, substantially limited his ability to work (it also ruled that his employer could fire him to save money—especially on health insurance).

Similarly, Boyle, with his leukemia in remission, sued the Texas company for which he worked twenty years when he was demoted from president to vice president. The court rejected his case, holding that the "only limitation that Boyle identified was his need to take time off for chemotherapy [over a six-month period; each treatment lasted from three to five days]. That need is not a disability under the act."

These cases, wrote Hoffman, drive home three lessons crucial to winning a case under the ADA:

1. You must show exactly *how* either your cancer or its treatment limited a major life activity, or show that your employer thought your cancer limited a major life activity. Don't assume the court—or for that matter, your attorney—understands cancer or its impact on you.
2. You should file a claim under each definition of disability in the ADA (you have a disability, a history of a disability, or your employer regarded your cancer as a disability) for which you have any supporting evidence.
3. You must show that your employer treated you differently *because* of your cancer diagnosis. Courts will look at the timing of when your employer learned you had cancer and when it acted against you, the employer's credibility, and how the employer treated other workers.

Cancer disability advocates emphasize that survivors facing discrimination should pause and think before they sue. Such men and women, say the experts, should let their employers know they are aware of their legal rights and would rather resolve the issues openly and honestly than file a lawsuit (which might drag on a long time and prove expensive). Such informal discussions often result in accommodations suitable to both parties—arranging, for example, to work extra hours on the days you do not have chemotherapy.

Caveats: survivors should be careful of what they say during such discussions so that they do not hurt their claim should they later decide to take formal action. And they should keep carefully written records of all job actions, both good and bad.

A survey done in 1996 highlighted the formidable amount of education still needed at century's end—for employers and their staffs, survivors, judges, and, yes, even attorneys and the public at large. It revealed that although four out of five cancer survivors (81 percent of the five hundred interviewed) felt their job helped them maintain emotional stability while undergoing treatment, they were at five times higher risk for firings and lay-offs than other American workers.

Importantly, the survey, sponsored by the biotechnical company Amgen and *Working Woman* magazine, questioned significant numbers of supervisors and co-workers, as well as survivors employed at the time of treatment. Of the two hundred supervisors interviewed, 33 percent believed that the survivors could *not* handle both the job and cancer, and 31 percent thought the employee needed to be replaced. But after working with a survivor, 34 percent of the supervisors and 43 percent of the co-workers said that they would be less concerned about working with a survivor in the future.

Leafing through *Bartlett's* the other day, I came across Angela Morgan's stirring vision of the human need to work. For me, her words summed it up:

> Work!
> Thank God for the swing of it,
> For the clamoring, hammering ring of it,
> Passion of labor daily hurled
> On the mighty anvils of the world.

Clearly, a good many subtle factors enter into workplace attitudes and decisions that deter survivors from hurling their passion for labor on the world's mighty anvils, according to his or her own personhood and dreams.

Some employers worry about the psychological impact of a survivor's cancer history on other employees. Others fail to revise their personnel policies to comply with new laws or have not trained their personnel properly. And, as we shall see in the next chapter, economic factors—like possible increased insurance costs or reduced productivity—still drive a good part of what happens to survivors in the workplace.

11 ❧ *Money*

At first glance, this support group at D.C. General Hospital—our capital's "hospital of last resort," which treats all comers, regardless of ability to pay—resembles many I have visited during my long cancer journey. It meets twice a month, on Wednesday mornings, behind an outpatient clinic in a stuffy, windowless room around a long table; a blackboard leaves chalked traces of other meetings ("We appreciate our social workers—The Nurses"). Various members (women usually; though men are welcome, few attend) bring friendly offerings of juice and cookies to each meeting. Led and encouraged by two social workers, the two-hour sessions can go slowly but pick up when one of the middle-aged, largely African American patients with one or another kind of cancer strikes a common nerve.

And that nerve often leads—either directly or indirectly—to money and what money buys in the way of knowledge, habits, and lifestyle. Ruth Ann Hackley, a breast cancer survivor who also suffers from Crohn's disease (she has had a colostomy) and asthma, strikes that nerve when she starts to talk about being on "spend down" (under the federal-state Medicaid program for low-income Americans, when your income is above a certain level, you have to "spend down" to get financial help, letting your bills accumulate and getting rid of any extra "nonessentials," like a car). The other women chime in; most have been on and off "spend down." They have to worry not only about their cancer and often a host of other conditions but also how to find and hold on to insurance or some other means of paying for their health care.

Listen to them and you will hear how, when they first came to this hospital (on whose governing commission I once served) with its now $152 million annual budget, they paid a $20 registration fee. Then, with the considerable help of hospital social workers and financial counselors, they and their families struggled to put together a patchwork of public and occasional private programs that would pay for their care. Not an easy job.

The paperwork involved in qualifying for Medicaid is formidable (some 47 percent of D.C. General's bills are covered by this federal-state insurance, with its good benefits but stringent categories and regulations, or by the federal Medicare program for patients sixty-five and over; a significant portion of the rest is picked up by the District government's Medical Charities subsidy; only a tiny percentage is covered by private insurance). And, especially when you've been sick and do not have a family to help out, running around downtown from office to office to get that paperwork processed can be both demanding and exhausting. Understandably, these survivors feel wary of questions and forms (for that reason their names are changed here).

Beyond that, the problems that so often accompany cancer— the difficulty of finding transportation to get to medical treatment, to get out to enjoy life a bit more, the feelings of loneliness and fatigue and not understanding what the (possibly foreign-born) doctor is telling you—are all exaggerated when you are poor. "I'm telling you my body has never seen such changes," says Ronnie Jackson. "It's like a yo-yo. One minute I'm hurting, one minute I'm not. And I want to cling to the bed and just sleep. But I try not to do that because that's bad."

Lara Joynes nods. Her isolation is more acute since she and her husband have moved into a new neighborhood. A tall, sharp-looking woman in white duck pants and a flowered shirt, she has learned new makeup tricks from a Look Good . . . Feel Better cosmetologist who comes to the hospital (an American Cancer Society program). Since her laryngectomy, she has had a hard time talking; but with speech therapy, she has made good

progress and suggests that Ruth Ann can get the new wig she
wants from that same program. Social worker Jacqueline Downing asks Ruth Ann if she might want that.

Ruth Ann, nods, gratefully. A new wig from Downing might
help her more than the mental health clinic she consults
(because of the crying spells she has suffered). Not only does she
want to look and feel better, but she worries that she delayed
bringing her breast tumor to medical attention, while her bra
increased in size. She hungers for information. "My doctor don't
tell me a thing about all my pills," she explains. "And I've got a
lot wrong with me." Diana Ames agrees. "I want to learn as
much as possible. If you know about it, if you talk about it,
you're not scared. I was coming to this hospital for tension;
when I got breast cancer I found out I had diabetes too. In case it
happens to me, I want to know about it."

If you know about it, if you talk about it, you're not scared.
Social worker Amy Monteiro announces that a pharmacist will
come to the group to discuss the members' medicines and
answer questions. She passes around a newspaper clipping about
T'ai Chi—nice, relaxing stretching exercises they can do for
stress. A T'ai Chi teacher has worked with the group and will
return. Downing explains that the group survivors feel comfortable here at D.C. General in familiar surroundings. "The Lord
did bless me," adds Louise Jackson. "I'm right around the corner
from this hospital." She reports that at first she thought she did
not need a support group. But her family had never experienced
cancer; they could not relate to her in her new state. "So I called
and tried to find a group close to me and they gave me one
that was held at night—in an area that's a war zone at night; I
wouldn't be caught over there."

A few seem a bit defensive of D.C. General, a teaching hospital for several area medical schools. "We get doctors from How-
ard and Georgetown and even Johns Hopkins here," Diane Ames
proudly tells skeptical friends. But they are glad that this institution, which has been through some hard times and recently
became part of a quasi-public corporation (including referring
public health clinics), has survived and earned high marks in its
latest official reaccreditation survey. They do not lack for state-

of-the-art cancer care (like a five-year course of adjuvant chemotherapy to prevent the recurrence of breast cancer or speech
therapy after a laryngectomy). Still, if one needed special ter-
tiary care (say, open-heart surgery), he or she would have a
harder time.

And they have their own support group impossible to con-
ceive of when I served this 150-year-old hospital in the late
1970s and 1980s—in a relatively new Ambulatory Care building then only a gleam in the commission's eyes. Through the
group, they are making new friends and gaining support that
has empowered them. ("Tell me *your* story," says Lara when I
ask her hers. I do.) Between meetings, they often call each other
for information and encouragement.

At meeting's end we are discussing—of all things—the uncomfortable constipation our medicines frequently cause.
"Heat your prune juice," advises one of the women.

Downing tells Lara that she will help her find a "little program near you—perhaps at a church or with the AARP. One I
know takes people for trips and to theatre."

Silence. "It's only $4 a ticket," explains the social worker.
"And it's good to get out. One *must* get out."

We are all *out*. We stand with our arms crossed, holding
hands, as she leads us in a closing prayer.

Since then, I have been drinking hot prune juice. And thinking
about money and its effect on survivors, of all income levels,
cultures, and persuasions. Out of the theories and statistics that
address this complicated subject, I can conclude only one thing:
despite great changes in our nation's way of managing health
care in the past decades, money remains the paper anomaly of
the survivor culture, king in an economic never-never land. It
reigns all important yet often singularly unimportant, unreal,
yet real enough to affect the subtlest part of our lives. For
money, or more broadly, what money buys in the way of habits
and lifestyle, seems to affect both who gets cancer in the first
place (incidence) and how we do after we get it (survival).

Studies of cancer incidence are maddeningly complex and
difficult to sort out; you can only glean clues from them as to

cause and effect. But researchers have been finding for some
time that certain population groups suffer more cancer than others and suffer it in different ways. Since such groups in our plu-
ralistic society often have different average income levels and
different styles in which they use that income, the implication,
at least, is that income is involved in disease incidence.

When the National Cancer Institute and Centers for Disease
Control and Prevention, along with the American Cancer Society,
announced in early 1998 that, after almost twenty years of steady
increase, both the number of new cancer cases in the United
States (cancer incidence) and the death rate were dropping, the
news was greeted with joy. And considerable caution, particularly
on the part of minority survivor leaders like Zora Brown (founder
and head of the Breast Cancer Resource Committee, which works
with African American women). They were quick to point out
that there were dark spots in this rosier picture.

For the new statistics comparing the periods 1973 to 1990 and
1990 to 1995 showed again that cancer strikes unfairly. Looking
at incidence rates for each of the four leading cancer sites—
accounting for 54 percent of newly diagnosed cancers of the lung
and bronchus, prostate, female breast, and colon/rectum—one
saw that, except for breast cancer, blacks had higher incidence
rates than whites, Asians and Pacific Islanders, or Hispanics.
Moreover, black women suffered higher breast cancer mortality
rates than other groups of women; black men had the highest
cancer rates of any group, mainly because of a sharp rise in new
cases of prostate cancer.

In the same way, decreases in the incidence of some cancers
among blacks occurred later than among whites. Although the
earliest decreases in incidence occurred for male lung cancer in
both whites and blacks in the mid-1980s, decreases among
blacks generally came later than among whites—beginning for
colon/rectum cancer for whites in the mid-1980s and in blacks
not until the early 1990s. Decreases in prostate cancer in
blacks appeared to begin in the mid-1990s, in contrast to the
early 1990s for whites.

Various experts attributed the decline in new cases to changes
in behavior—notably a drop in smoking—and the decline in deaths

to increased screening and better therapies. Looking at it another way, some explained that such advances do not affect Americans equally because minorities are less likely to be screened, less likely to have cancer detected early, and less likely to get the best therapy; this, in turn, might be due to low levels of income and lower likelihood of health insurance coverage.

Combing through a bunch of recent research papers (which, one must remember, usually take several years to work their way through the review and publication process), I concluded that the studies ascribing cancer incidence and survival differences to socioeconomic status (SES), and particularly to the neighborhoods in which people lived, made particular sense. Nancy Breen, Ph.D., and Martin L. Brown, Ph.D., researchers based at the National Cancer Institute, are among those who have shown that living in a socially disadvantaged or "underserved" neighborhood is a strong predictor of invasive cancer. Living in a neighborhood with a high proportion of households in poverty is also a strong predictor.

In such neighborhoods, people are likely to have more trouble accessing hospitals and clinics, as well as finding doctors who accept lower Medicaid reimbursement rates, and transportation to them. They also may delay cancer screening and diagnosis. And, without help, they often lack the know-how to deal with such health problems as a multiplicity of diseases (co-morbidity, in scientific lingo). The women in our D.C. General support group personify the fact that African American women with breast cancer are more likely than white women to have another disease and twice as likely to have two other diseases. And I have learned at several of the "Minorities, the Medically Underserved, and Cancer" symposia how aggrieved are Hispanic Americans as, for example, they report that cervical cancer rates among Hispanic American women are the highest of any minority group, except for Vietnamese women. Or that only 70 percent of Hispanic women diagnosed with breast cancer survive longer than five years, compared with 84 percent of the Caucasian population.

But though money and insurance help determine access, and access itself is critical, it does not account completely for the

extra cancer burden suffered by minorities. At the 1997 symposium, Martha Spinks, an army social worker, explained why
cultural background and even physical differences often have
to be considered. "Are Racial Differences in [Breast Cancer] Survival Explained by Access to Medical Care?" she asked, and her
answer, produced by a study of more than sixty-five hundred
army spouses and other women (10 percent of them black), was,
unexpectedly, "No."

African Americans and whites receive equal access to treatment in the Department of Defense health care system. And
though the African American beneficiaries fared much better
than those in the general population, there were still significant
differences in survival between black and white women that
may be due to differences in biology (notably in reproductive
history and obesity), cultural factors (diet or perception of the
health care system), or socioeconomic characteristics (environmental hazards or opportunity for preventive health measures).

So we see that the role of money in cancer incidence can be
fuzzy. It becomes somewhat clearer when it comes to what happens to you after you are diagnosed with cancer.

Most obvious: the cancer we band of sisters—and brothers—
suffer is a very expensive disease. Our bills are big, and someone,
some entity, whether it be individual or group, taxpayer or private charity, must pick them up. The person who is not insured—
either publicly or privately, against what economists call "direct
costs," or the costs of our medical care and treatment—is in sorry
straits.

Direct costs vary, of course, depending on what kind of cancer
you are measuring, its location, severity, and length of treatment. It is estimated that these costs account for more than
10 percent of our national medical bill and run annually into
the billions of dollars.

Until recently, individual direct costs have been calculated
on a yearly basis—some two decades ago, for example, we estimated my aggregated medical bills at around $11,000 a year.
Now experts are beginning to estimate the total, long-term cost
of our cancers—which makes sense, looking at it from a national,

public health, not a personal or family, point of view. At the lower end of the scale, a group at a cost-conscious health maintenance organization (HMO), Kaiser Permanente of Northern California, estimated the cost from diagnosis until death or fifteen years this way: breast, $35,000; colon, $42,000; rectum, $51,000; lung, $31,000; ovarian, $64,000; prostate, $29,000; and non-Hodgkin's lymphoma, $48,000.

These big bucks estimates are likely to be even higher in other settings. The breast cancer treatment I—and most of the women in the D.C. General group—have suffered is estimated by the American Association for Cancer Research (AACR) to cost the United States about $10 billion a year and to add $5,000 a year to the health care costs of the average American woman. According to the AACR, this disease costs some $55,000, rather than $35,000, per patient, while local treatments for prostate cancer, including surgery and radiation, can cost between $10,000 and $20,000, and the cost to treat advanced disease can range from $30,000 to $100,000. Similarly, the $20,000 to $40,000 cost of treatment for head and neck cancer can be enhanced by specialized reconstructive surgery costing $10,000 to $20,000—not to speak of the added costs for psychosocial treatment for the human problems involved.

Such estimates do not even cover the "direct" costs of nonstandard, often "experimental" treatments like extremely aggressive high-dose chemotherapy and/or bone marrow transplants (which can run $100,000–$150,000 and are frequently and unfortunately inaccessible, even to insured survivors). And of smaller but important out-of-pocket extras like transportation to treatment (including such items as bridge or tunnel tolls, parking fees, gasoline, or bus fare), extra help around the house, and child care during it. Nor the "indirect costs" of loss of employment, job promotion or improvement, or even leisure time or volunteer activities.

When I present myself (often without breakfast) for a scan, or another test, or an outpatient biopsy at a hospital or medical center clinic desk, the admitting personnel do not even say "good morning." They do not ask for money, directly.

Instead, they ask, "May I see your insurance cards?" And when I increasingly have to pay cash out of pocket for at least part of a pricey oral medication I take these days, I am surprised. Again, after the patients arriving at D.C. General pay their twenty-dollar registration fee, they are involved more in filling out the appropriate forms than shelling out cash for medical care.

This is because the medical marketplace differs from any other. Traditionally, buyers and sellers of health care seldom faced each other at the cash register or even discussed cost. Unaccustomed to customers' reaching into their wallets, counting their bills, and paying for a health service or product directly, both have tended to be less sensitive to the price of health care than they were during the sale of anything else probably less essential to human well-being, such as a new car or a newfangled computer.

Everyone knew that someone else—some third party in an insurance or government office—would pay the bill, not out of goodness of the heart, but because the buyers, as individuals and taxpayers, had over the years prepaid through insurance plans, and the plans paid the bills wherever they used services. In such an unconstrained *fee-for-service system,* we signed forms documenting doctor or hospital use; medical offices fed items about our care first into metal files and, in modern times, into computers.

Eventually we received either a bill or reams of incomprehensible computer printouts. If we were lucky and had enough time, we might be able to figure out what we owed and to whom, and what part of our costs insurance would pay. Such a marketplace drove medical costs skyward (a 12 percent annual increase in the 1980s translated into a 90 percent leap in insurance premiums between 1987 and 1993). Consequently, the larger society intervened: in the 1980s, the federal government tried to control costs (by capping certain of them); in the 1990s it also tried to "reform" the system, or nonsystem—with little success—and the nation's employers, who footed much of the bill, stepped in at least to help control the costs.

The result, at century's end, is a diffuse medical marketplace in a state of flux—where new kinds of health care delivery organizations have developed, usually involving specific providers and charging an enrolled population a fixed yearly fee rather than billing members for care each time they become ill. Aiming to control costs, increase the efficiency of care, and particularly to minimize the need for expensive inpatient hospitalization, these new organizations have taken over an increasing share of the marketplace. Most of their insurance plans are offered by employers to their employees in the workplace, giving these consumers—as long as they work in large organizations and enjoy good health—the option to be cost- as well as benefit-conscious as they select providers and use services. For some consumers, the advantages of broader benefits—including immunizations, physicals, and other preventive services—and the promise of lower costs outweigh the hassles of a limited choice and an often irritating set of rules to getting care.

Some 60 to 70 percent of Americans under sixty-five years of age have enrolled in these *managed care* groups—most profit-making, a minority nonprofit, some with physicians working in a group under one roof (HMOs), others using doctors with individual practices (preferred provider organizations, or PPOs), some sponsored by private, some by public sector entities, some restricting provider choice, others allowing enrollees to use all health providers or institutions in their network but also to go outside it for services for an additional fee.

In the mushrooming of such new systems, money had become much more visible and costs more central. Still, our aspirations for the newest, the best that modern medicine offers remain sky high; if new, even esoteric treatments take shape, we want them, we *will* have them, no matter the cost. But no law guarantees that all cancer survivors, or anyone else, can buy even adequate affordable health care. As Professor Judith Feder of Georgetown University's Public Policy Institute (now dean of policy studies at Georgetown) points out, getting that affordable care has become a formidable problem.

The bulk of this problem, according to Feder, has to do with the fact that "people who don't have health coverage cannot afford it—either employers do not offer it to them or the premiums are too high; only a minority are unemployed." Lesser problems have to do with a certain "innocence" of the crucial need for health insurance coverage. This is seen particularly in young people who have flown the protective parental nest feeling well, strong, and invulnerable, says Irene Card, a New Jersey health insurance claims specialist. Irene, who has worked diligently with the National Coalition for Cancer Survivorship (NCCS) over the years to help people who cannot afford coverage find ways of paying for medical care, reports that such young people come to her astounded to find themselves up the creek, ill with cancer and uninsured.

But their number is small compared with those who are struggling for adequate coverage in today's medical marketplace. Like many other financial counselors working with cancer patients, Irene Card reserves her particular scorn for the managed care system whose rules, regulations, and cost-saving approach can threaten survivors of all ages who thought they were protected. One HMO, she reports, planned to send a client of hers three thousand miles away from home for a bone marrow transplant because it was cheaper. Another allowed a survivor to become strangled by rules that kept him from getting permission from his primary physician-"gatekeeper" to travel to M. D. Anderson Cancer Center in Texas to consult a specialist. Still others keep stalling on providing a badly needed transplant considered experimental until the survivor dies.

True, there are HMOs and HMOs—some managed care organizations offer only bare-bones care or ways of dealing with doctors and hospitals, while others stretch themselves to provide quality care even as they stabilize costs. At least one large study of 13,358 women with breast cancer in the San Francisco–Oakland and Seattle–Puget Sound areas showed that long-term survival outcomes in two prepaid group practice HMOs were at least equal to, and possibly better than, outcomes in the fee-for-service system (and more frequently used recommended breast-conserving surgery and radiotherapy for early-stage breast cancer).

Beyond that, in a competitive system, some innovative managed care models offer a combination of case management, social services, counseling, rehabilitation, and more to cancer

survivors, along with more mundane services like valet parking
and improved, even tasty hospital food service.

Still, managed care—which some call "mangled" or "misman-
aged" care—had irritated enough Americans by the end of the
1990s to become, as one headline writer put it, a "hot political
issue." This became clear to me, of all places, at the movies,
about halfway through a showing of *As Good As It Gets*. A roar
of empathetic approval went up from the audience when a New
York waitress blasted her HMO in pretty stiff language. The reason: the waitress's ogre of a health plan wouldn't let her get
the proper care for her severely asthmatic son. The boy gasps for
breath on the ride to the hospital; the film audience feels his and
his mother's pain.

No matter that this single parent waitress-mom was at least
insured, that other quality-minded HMOs (which, of course,
might not have been available to the waitress through her small
employer) might have managed his disease more efficiently even
while controlling overall costs, preventing the child's ever
reaching an asthmatic crisis. *As Good As It Gets* had struck a
nerve; children, pragmatic Americans feel, simply should not
suffer because money has become a higher priority than quality
health care on some big bureaucrat's agenda.

No wonder that members of both major political parties—
particularly those who are running for election and reelection—
call for a sweeping "patients' bill of rights" that would give
consumers more weapons in dealing with their managed care
organizations, like the right to appeal decisions or choose
their own doctors and specialists.

If, at century's end, money had become more visible at the ful-
crum of health care change, it still occupied a peculiar, evanes-
cent place in the hanging-in cancer culture: now you see it, now
you don't.

The majority of Americans who are insured in some way
against major costs and preoccupied with their own problems
can forget a crucial fact: many of us are not even insured.
According to the U.S. Census Bureau, an estimated 43.4 million
people—16 percent of the population—had no health insurance

during the entire 1997 calendar year. And this was up from 41.7 million in 1996. Some experts hold that since roughly 60 percent of cancer survivors are aged sixty-five or more (see chapter 5), they are less likely to fall within this uninsured group than other disease survivors, because they are entitled to Medicare—which, with its many holes for those who cannot afford supplemental or Medigap coverage for noncovered costs, is still insurance.

Survivor activists counter that since most adults obtain health insurance through their employment, any cancer-connected loss of employment increases the risk of lost or decreased coverage among working-aged men and women. And they stress that the psychological costs—the costs in human suffering—if you are without insurance can only be imagined, for they have been scantily studied.

Even underinsured survivors can be seriously distressed, according to social worker Myra Glajchen, former director of research for Cancer Care who is now the director of education at Beth Israel Medical Center in New York City. Studying a group of 187 ambulatory care patients, virtually all of whom had some type of health insurance, she found that patients with more coverage and more than one insurance provider (such as Medicare and Blue Cross/Blue Shield) reported less psychological distress, less financial burden, and reduced concern about that burden than those with less coverage and fewer insurance providers.

What's more, 67 percent of the group indicated that problems with health insurance and cost had affected their medical decision making—especially in terms of staying in a job to maintain coverage and selecting a physician covered by their insurance plan. And significant numbers had to change their lifestyles and spend savings to offset financial burdens (like co-payments, deductibles, premiums, and expenses not covered by insurance).

Still, most of us lucky, fully covered survivors do not see money exchanged too much from day to day—though we are beginning to see it more. I do not see it when I visit my oncologist for a cancer check-up and never even look at my pink patient/insurance copy of the form handed me recording my status as an "established patient," my diagnoses, and the cost of the

visit. I simply fold it and put it in my handbag—as I would a form
acknowledging service from a surgeon or hospital—knowing
that as a fee-for-service Medicare patient with a good (though
increasingly expensive) Medigap policy, I do not have to worry
about incredibly expensive out-of-pocket health care expenses
(except for dental bills).

I do see it speaking to a group of American Association of
Retired Persons (AARP) volunteers working on breast cancer
issues at an AARP meeting in California. Having just heard NBC
doctor/guru Art Ulene advise us to use our Medicare cards to
reward providers of choice with our business, I asked members
of the audience to stand if they, like me, had been turned away
by doctors (often specialists) because of their status as Medicare
patients (for whose care physicians are reimbursed at a lower
rate). Responding eagerly, fully a third—perhaps half—of the large
audience stood up. Like me, they had been told by Medicare-shy
doctors that they would have to pay full (way higher than Medicare) rates by check or cash—up front—if they wanted an appointment. (Most cannot afford such an offer even if they find it
acceptable. Some people's solution—just letting us pay extra
for special access—may work for a few, but it would destroy complete protection for the majority.)

Again, money was only dimly visible to one survivor when
her Iowa HMO not only treated her breast cancer successfully
but also arranged for an ensuing heart transplant without any
ifs, ands, or buts. Objecting to HMO-bashing, she rose at a recent
National Breast Cancer Coalition (NBCC) conference session on
managed care to insist she would not be standing there alive and
kicking without an HMO that went all out for her when she
needed it.

But it was all too visible when I read in the *New York Times*
how an insurance company based in the same state of Iowa
denied twenty-nine-year-old melanoma survivor Michael
Mulloy treatment with high-dose chemotherapy with stem
cell rescue that it considered "experimental." Outraged, Mulloy's Sloan-Kettering physician in New York City argued that
neither the drug nor the treatment was experimental and that it
was the young man's last chance for a meaningful period of sur-

vival. Refusing to pay, a company representative told the patient
to hold a fund-raiser.

People in other industrialized countries who enjoy some sort of
"universal health care" (where everyone is insured) often fail to
understand our way of assuring—or trying to assure—health care.
At NCCS assemblies, our Canadian colleagues have been bewil-
dered to hear our stories of difficulties in getting and staying
adequately insured; their bills, on leaving the hospital after a
cancer episode, usually amount to less than ten dollars for television service or spouse parking fees.

Preparing to give Hope & Cope's annual lecture in Montreal,
Canada, in the fall of 1998, I wrote that group's executive director asking about the issues of greatest interest to my prospective
audience. I both laughed and cried when I read her response:
since Canadian survivors "do *not* have issues of insurance/
employer discrimination and access to health care as you have
in the U.S.," the group would be more concerned with psychosocial concerns than advocacy issues. Laughed—because our
northern neighbors are lucky enough to enjoy a situation in
which no one is ever refused health care (and cancer is accorded
special priority). Cried—because we are not.

That said, I must add that at century's end, in Canada as in
the States, health care resources are stretched, people are paying
more out of pocket for health care, and short waits for radiation
treatment because of a shortage of radiation oncologists have
increased. In addition, as in the States, people with money have
more options and fare better than those who have less. Still, universal coverage is the order of the day.

Once, when I was abroad interviewing a Spanish health
official, I mentioned that we had no one comprehensive health
plan similar to those in European countries, which, despite their
problems, cover everyone. I explained that we had such programs only for older Americans and for the very poor. He did not
believe me. Surely such a situation could not prevail in the land
of milk, honey, brain scans, computer chips, and the best health
care in the world! "What?" he asked, appalled. "Not even in the
District of California? Not even in the District of Illinois?"

Not even in the District of California. Not even in the District of Illinois. Our society has often produced extraordinary and effective therapies that have prolonged cancer survival, but we have not provided a way to ensure them adequately for all survivors. Having failed to achieve some sort of national health care reform in the early 1990s, we continue to chip away at the task. The 1996 Health Insurance Portability and Accountability Act (or "Kassebaum-Kennedy" law), for instance, has protected survivors caught in infamous "job lock" situations. To a certain extent.

Take my friend Anna Wu Work, Ph.D., a molecular biologist, who hit the front page of the *New York Times* in 1991 when she found herself afraid to leave her job as a full-time researcher at a Los Angeles hospital or to ask for part-time work so she could spend more time with her two young daughters. The reason: three years earlier she had suffered early-stage breast cancer and thus had a "previously existing condition" threatening to prospective insurers. She remembers that she and her cardiologist husband "were a young couple in the early stages of our career, early stages of our marriage, early stages of our family, with such grand plans!" Then cancer intervened, and they could not find the insurance they felt they needed, in the unlikely event of recurrence of her breast cancer.

Today, Anna would be able to change jobs if she wished (she does not) because the Health Insurance Portability and Accountability Act will not generally allow insurers to deny coverage (if employers offer it) because of "previously existing conditions" (and in several other ways it increases insurance portability from group to group or group to individual plans). But it does not provide all survivors with the means to buy it, and, in the open market, such insurance can prove expensive. Anna, although she probably could afford this expense now, remembers how differently she and her husband had acted at the time of her diagnosis—"not as alert or aware as we are now." That is why she volunteers, as a scientist/faculty member of the NBCC's project LEAD (Leadership, Education, and Advocacy Development), to teach others about the science of breast cancer and the issues surrounding it.

Survivors can fall between the cracks in many other ways, as well. I always get a nervous laugh from audiences when I cite "marriage lock," a laugh that betrays familiarity with a situation more intimate but no less real than "job lock"—wherein survivors are locked into unhappy marriages that provide them with indispensable health insurance plans they cannot afford on their own.

More tangibly, others in need of care find themselves too young for Medicare or, like a puzzled member of the D.C. General group who works for a cleaning service, "making too much money to get on Medicaid" (or unable for some other reason to fit into one of that program's stringent eligibility categories). Or, even if they are older and qualified for Medicare, unable to afford a pricey "Medigap" policy to supplement it. Or working for a small business that cannot afford to cover them. Or self-employed and simply priced out of the health care market.

Or they may simply be unaware of their vulnerability. At a press conference held at the Johns Hopkins Hospital because "I don't want anybody to be as dumb as I was," longtime Maryland activist and now cancer survivor Bea Gaddy wept as she confessed she had never thought cancer would happen to her. She had found uncounted hours to help others find food and shelter, the *Baltimore Sun* reported, but never time to find the coverage and so the preventive screening she now urged for others.

Health policy experts describe those who seek somehow to find insurance protection as "running for cover," and they advise uncovered people, if they are working age, to get a job, any job in which they would be eligible for group insurance coverage (it's not likely that you would be able to afford individual insurance now anyway, particularly if you are already sick). Put your pride on the shelf, they say. The job itself—with a temporary office help firm, for instance—is not your goal; it's the health coverage that job brings with it.

If you cannot work even part-time, they continue, check to see whether any organizations or associations you belong to or could belong to offer group health insurance plans. Some professional and fraternal organizations, alumni/ae organizations or groups such as the National Association for the Self-Employed or state insurance commissioners, can steer you in the direction in which you want to go.

In this confused environment, in which all health care has become "managed" to some degree and patient options often turn out to be much more theoretical and limited than initially supposed, *quality*, as much as money, has become the name of the game. Once the health powers that be, in government, in private industry, in the health system itself, had begun to contain health dollars, they turned their attention to the quality of what those dollars purchased—to, as the National Academy of Science's Institute of Medicine defined it, "the degree to which health services for individuals and populations increase the likelihood of desired health outcomes and are consistent with current professional knowledge."

For us survivors, as for other health care consumers, this was a whole new ball game. As employers who purchase health plans for employees, and health industry managers who compete for their business, and government officials responsible for public health programming had become more interested in the quality as well as the cost of care, everyone seemed to have questions for us:

What did we think of our care? Why had we made certain choices between different services? Were different managed care organizations or individual doctors and hospitals delivering quality care? Or was such care being denied or otherwise stymied in the interest of greater financial return? Were insurers being held *accountable* (another new buzzword) for quality care and the way it was delivered? Had we found, as many had, that quality varied within the United States from place to place and doctor to doctor? (A woman on Medicare who is diagnosed with breast cancer in Elyria, Ohio, for instance, is thirty-three times more likely to have breast-conserving surgery instead of mastectomy than a woman in Rapid City, South Dakota.)

Though most of us were not medically trained (and usually had little interest in going to medical school), we had to learn not just whether and why we "liked" certain doctors and health plans but the difference between the quality and nonquality services they delivered and so how to select one, rather than another. To do so, we needed information—in spades. And this need, along with the needs of health care officialdom wanting more bang for its health care buck, led to a major effort to refine the process of measuring, comparing, and reporting on the quality as well as the price of care.

No easy task. For one thing, there is, thus far, no federal requirement for health plans to collect and report standardized data. For another, not all doctors and hospitals really wanted their work measured. Even some of those who do want their services measured so as to improve their practices do not always know how to go about it. Many, for instance, had long used "consumer satisfaction surveys" to supplement such tools as utilization review in measuring care. It seemed hard for them to switch gears and find ways of quantifying, not numbers of patients seen, or specialist referrals, or even time spent in waiting rooms, but the overall quality of care they offered, including the outcomes of that care and the degree of patient trust they enjoyed.

At one medical center advisory committee meeting, a group of cancer center administrators were puzzled at the results of a survey I had participated in as a patient, which showed high patient satisfaction with our doctors but only lukewarm approval of their care. How, they wanted to know, could such a dichotomy exist?

"Easily," I told them, and I explained that though the survivors loved their doctors, the cancer center clinic had not earned their trust: they did not love not having their questions about biopsy results answered in timely fashion, for example. Or being treated at the admissions desk, not like human beings, but like run-of-the-mill "cases." They did not like the clumsy way their veins had, at times, been punctured in the lab by careless technicians.

In the mid- and late 1990s, new tools were forthcoming whereby quality and accountability could be measured and compared. Of these, perhaps the best known were the "report cards" issued by the National Committee for Quality Assurance (NCQA). This private nonprofit group started largely by big employers and managed care companies (but now with a more representative board) evaluates managed care plans for accreditation. But its measurement system, or HEDIS (Health Plan Employer Data and Information Set), was skewed to measure the processes used by a health plan to provide care—how effectively it works to improve its care, for example, or investigates its physicians' qualification and practice history, or uses preventive services like immunizations and mammograms—and not to set standards for outcomes or consumer satisfaction with those outcomes.

Because it is not a regulatory agency, the NCQA cannot take action against plans that do not meet its standards, but many employers and organizations use its scorecard in deciding which plans to offer. To date only 167 out of the 281 plans reviewed (there are a total of 650 plans) have been fully accredited, with 12 being denied outright.

The nonprofit Foundation for Accountability (FACCT), based in Portland, Oregon, focuses more completely on us—the health care users. With a board that from the beginning included consumers as well as government and big corporate purchasers, FACCT is dedicated to creating quality measurement and reporting tools that reflect our needs. Such quality measurement sets, which have been applied to breast cancer and a number of other conditions (including adult asthma, diabetes, and depression), tell consumers how well the health care system performs in five areas:

> *The basics.* Delivering the basics of good care—doctor care, rules for getting care, information and service, satisfaction;
> *Staying healthy.* Helping people avoid illness and stay healthy through preventive care, reduction of health risks, early detection of illness, education;
> *Getting better.* Helping people recover when they're sick or injured through appropriate treatment and follow up;
> *Living with illness.* Helping people with ongoing, chronic conditions take care of themselves, control symptoms, avoid complications, and maintain daily activities;

Changing needs. Caring for people and their families when needs change dramatically because of disability or terminal illness—with comprehensive services, caregiver support, hospice care.

Other groups, such as the federal Agency for Health Care Policy and Research (AHCPR), are working to develop evidence-based clinical guidelines that will help in practitioner and patient decision making (particularly hard in oncology, with its large variety of cancers and diverse population of diagnosed patients). The results of all these efforts will be more accessible to survivors as private and public employers, as well as publications like *Consumer Reports,* publish "report cards" on competing plans (the federal government's Medicare+Choice program now has an online database to help consumers chose between different plans)—and as consumer networks publicize them.

But it's well to keep in mind that all the information in the world, and all the rights to use it in making medical choices, can be useless if you are underinsured or if you have no health coverage at all.

Without coverage, or without adequate coverage, *quality* becomes an empty word. Your cancer may not even be discovered. If it is, the probability is strong that your care will be suboptimal—surgery (if possible), and little more. And then, no one will be accountable for it. Even in absentia, money becomes highly visible.

12 ❧ *The Big Picture*
A Search for Meaning

To feel, to be alive. When Ivan Ilych, the hero of Tolstoy's great short story, lay dying, he listened to the voice of his own soul, to the current of thought rising within him.

"What do you want?" this voice asked. "What do you want?"

"What do I want? To live and not to suffer."

"To live? How?" asked his inner voice.

"Why to live as I used to, well and pleasantly."

"As you lived before, well and pleasantly?"

I had read and reread *The Death of Ivan Ilych* many times. In fact, I used that "to live and not to suffer" phrase repeatedly during my speech-writing days in the 1960s and 1970s, to encapsulate what patients want out of our health care system. That, alas, has not changed.

Until cancer entered my life, I never completely understood how Ivan, and his creator, Leo Tolstoy, felt as he lay on his couch, reviewing his life and seeking its meaning. Until then, like Ivan, I knew that "Caius is a man, men are mortal, therefore Caius is mortal." Like Ivan, I knew in the abstract that syllogism was true, "but certainly not as applied to himself" (myself).

Now, like other survivors in my position, I could no longer dismiss my own mortality. One day, perhaps sooner than later, I might not be alive. I could hope, I did hope, but my end would surely come. I had to ask myself: "What did it mean to die? To live? Was I making the best use of what time I had left?" Like many survivors described in this book, I felt a new sense of urgency when I developed cancer—particularly metastatic cancer. Death became more real to me. I knew I could never return to what author Susan Sontag has called "a more innocent relation to life."

Early on in my cancer journey, I remember telling my friend Nancy Harrison that perhaps I was spending too much time mulling over my situation. She had been hanging in much longer than I with breast cancer, and she told me that at the beginning she, too, often just sat on the couch weaving the psychic threads together, trying to figure it all out. Her husband had sometimes felt "enough's enough," but for her all the figuring-out hours were not time wasted. When her illness recurred, she became more and more active in her church, giving to her faith and gaining from it, cramming more and more into each day: one more church seminar, one more lecture, one more inner-city school project. Many felt this engaging woman, outstanding as she had been as a philanthropist and education leader, and successful as she had been as a wife and mother, was never so serene and fulfilled as in the last years of her life.

Over the years, I have been impressed with the number of survivors who grapple with spiritual concerns, particularly at the beginning and end of their cancer journeys—women and men who struggle to arrive at a more meaningful way of living each day as well as, finally, their last days. Last fall, on one of Cancer Care's helpful telephone conference calls (this one for some four hundred health care professionals, nationwide), I heard Mary Ellen Summerville, the organization's spirituality program coordinator, say that everyone has a human, spiritual dimension, though in some it is more developed than in others.

Patients and families struggle in different ways according to their backgrounds and beliefs, this social worker explained, not only with the possibility of imminent death, and the reality of eventual death (not necessarily from cancer, of course), but with issues of self-image: Do I lose value because I'm sick, bald, thin, unable to work or take care of my kids? Or do I have some enduring or inherent worth? And, importantly, issues of meaning: Why am I suffering? Is it because of something I did? Or is this just a random event? How can I make my life more meaningful now? Some ask if God is punishing them or using them in some way to show something to others or simply helping them through cancer.

Quoting experts like educator/psychologist Abraham Maslow, Mary Ellen spoke of society's, and particularly the helping professions', neglect, even denigration, of spiritual issues over much of the twentieth century, largely because of the schism between science and religion—with their respective turfs, the material world of matter and the body on the one hand, the spiritual and moral world on the other. I agreed with her feeling that this gap is beginning to close at the century's end, with each side gaining tolerance and respect for the other. As communication has exploded and the world has shrunk, *integration* has become the buzzword of the day—integration between the mind and the body (consider that confounding new discipline, psycho-neuroimmunology), integration between the holistic, peaceful, loving practices of the religions of distant, particularly Far Eastern, countries and those of our own (Yoga! Meditation! Deep breaths! Karma! Transcendent experiences!).

My interest was tweaked by her report of the small body of recent empirical research that has found an "overall association" between religious and spiritual belief and better-than-average mental and physical health. I had heard rumors of these findings at survivor meetings of one kind or another but had taken them with a grain of salt until I heard her references to such studies as one linking belief in God with higher self-esteem and another finding that cancer survivors with strong spiritual resources felt more sense that life is meaningful and suffered less depression, anxiety, or stress. A bit later a friend sent me a copy of a squib in a *Johns Hopkins Medical Letter* headed "Your faith may heal you," based on a review of empirical research published in the March-April 1998 *Archives of Family Medicine.* This article suggested—with the usual caveats such as "much remains to be investigated"—that religious commitment may "play a beneficial role" not only in preventing mental and physical illness but also in improving how people cope with such illness and in facilitating recovery.

Of course, not all cancer survivors can treat their experience as a challenge and use it to grow and find personal meaning and spiritual change. But if you can do so, it makes a difference. Former California chief justice Rose Elizabeth Bird has reported that after her first bout with cancer, she denied the possibility of recurrence and submerged herself in her work. Its recurrence was illuminating: "In a peculiar way," she told a Los Angeles medical forum, "death can teach you what life is all about. It is a painful lesson and a difficult journey, but I am personally grateful that I was made to travel this path at a relatively early age."

Her gratitude, this controversial jurist explained, stemmed from the increased time she had to learn much about herself, much about how precious life and people are to her, and to modify her behavior in various ways, so that she could, for example, eat in a more healthy way or try to deal more effectively with the stresses in her life. In short, she had time to do what the bishop in Margaret Craven's lyrical novel *I Heard the Owl Call My Name* told his young minister-protégé was the great benefit of living in the remote seacoast village of Kingcome, British Columbia, among the Kwakiutl Indians, where only the fundamentals count: to learn enough of the meaning of life to be ready to die.

In "Nourishing Our Spirits," one of a growing number of ecumenical "spirituality" groups, this one held at the Lombardi Cancer Center, I heard Suzanne, a tall, beautiful young woman with large hoop earrings, speak of how she had prayed for a child during years of marriage and finally had been blessed with a beautiful daughter—only to develop a virulent breast cancer. Why had her God blessed her so miraculously, only to turn about and cause her such pain? Puzzling this out took an inordinate amount of her precious time.

I responded that, similarly, I had once sat and stewed for long hours about my cancer predicament—my anxiety about my future, and possible lack of it, increasing. But as the months and then years went by and I gained self-confidence, I learned to stew less, to become more accepting and roll more agilely with the punches, trying to do the work (and play) I wanted to do, seeking emotional support when I needed it, and staying in touch with fellow survivors and others who made me feel upbeat and less afraid. I sometimes found such people where I least expected—at my longtime hairdresser's, for example, where my wobbling self-image was repeatedly restored (whether with hairpieces or other cosmetic coverups) by the supportive and skillful hands of Lucien et Eivind and their staff, who creatively and persistently repaired the ravages of treatment and the years it had added to my appearance.

The workaholic road suited me as it had the California justice. I threw myself into writing and consultant assignments as they came along. Though my first recurrence did not force a radical change, my second did cause me to examine my inchoate views of God and humankind and to reach some firmer convictions about the core of our existence. For me, this has taken a long time; I have come to assume the process (if that's what it is) will last as long as I do.

When I was still a "young" survivor at Sloan-Kettering in the 1970s, I wept as I talked to Sister Rosemary Moynihan, mourning the black hole, the nothingness of my newly found mortality. Back home, I floundered in my quest for answers to eternal riddles. It seemed to me that the strictly religious people were the fortunate ones. I envied their strong, clear faith, their ready access to language and symbols on which they could lean.

When she was told she had a good year to live, perhaps five or six more, with treatment, Marvella Bayh could ask with the old hymn, "Where could I go, but to the Lord?" She turned to her neighbor, a born-again Christian, for help in learning how to believe, to plug into God's healing love, to trust, to hope for a miracle, and to give her strength to further his work, through her own. Again, my hospital roommate, kerchief on her head and Medicaid card in her pocketbook, had far fewer earthly resources than I. But she had Jesus at her side, and she knew he was there, pitching for her. Similarly, my friend Nancy Harrison could forcefully challenge the young minister who was teaching the St. Alban's Church "Death" seminar she had organized when he dared to suggest that death might indeed be the end for us and that it was a mark of unselfish maturity to recognize and accept this. So strong was the opposition among those of our seminar mates who believed in some sort of resurrection, who were sure that an organized universe could not countenance lost souls, that the minister was made to retract his remarks at the next session, offering only a lame apology about the pressures in his life at the time.

But I was left, with him, uncertain and in doubt. I would have preferred to feel, like many men and women, that I would be rewarded in the next life if I endured suffering courageously, if I took up my cross with faith. Instead, I found myself a casualty of the traditional schism between science and religion, wondering if there was any concrete meaning in my pain. Turning to Reform Judaism, my own religion, I found myself in sync with the most skeptical of late biblical authors, Ecclesiastes, who applied his heart to know wisdom and concluded, "Whatsoever thy hand findeth to do, do it with all thy might; for there is no work, no device, nor knowledge, nor wisdom in Sheol [the grave], whither thou goest."

Ecclesiastes understood the search for meaning but warned off people like me who search too hard: "He hath made everything beautiful in its time," he tells us, "also he hath set eternity in their heart, yet so that man cannot find out the work that God hath done, from the beginning even to the end." That man—and woman—could not find out the work that God had done. Perhaps this is so; it remains a mystery, and I have grown more comfortable with that.

1977. My cancer had begun to metastasize; I called Bernard Mehlman, then rabbi of Temple Micah, the small teaching congregation to which we belong in Washington, and he came to my home within hours. We talked, I wept, and he recommended "The Heart Determines," Martin Buber's interpretation of Psalm 73. Later he sent me *Good and Evil*, the Buber book in which this essay appears, and said this had helped his sister in my same situation. I read and reread it, finding each time a reaffirmation of a suspicion: that our Bible, which exhorts us in such a magnificent way to choose life—the blessing rather than the curse—and would have us live it justly, mercifully, and humbly, offers us more abstruse, more complex understanding in death.

The essay, which seemed to me to reflect the thinking of Buber, the modern philosopher, as much as that of the biblical psalmist, explains that over against the realm of nothing, Sheol, there is God. The psalmist does not aspire to enter an empty heaven (for God's home is not there); nothing here implies being able to go into heaven after death ("And so far as I see," says Buber, "there is nowhere in the 'Old Testament' anything about this"). But he knows that in death he will have no desire to remain on earth, for now he will be wholly with Him who, like a guiding father, has grasped his hand and "'taken' him."

Here we have a different spin on what we are accustomed to calling personal immortality. The psalmist says, with what Buber calls "the strictest clarity," that it is not merely the flesh that vanishes in death but also his heart, the innermost personal organ of his soul, the seat of his imagination, and his rebelliousness (which can also be purified). Only the truest part of this person, the "rock" in which the heart is concealed—God—is eternal. Into His eternity moves he—and I must add she—who is pure in heart; this is something utterly different from any familiar mortal kind of time. "Separate souls vanish," Buber concludes. "Separation vanishes. Time which has been lived by the soul vanishes. . . . Existing man dies into eternity, as into the perfect existence."

My personal inquiry jagged off course a few years after my introduction to the Buber essay. My old friend and neighbor Hadassah, or "Handy," Davis dropped by during a visit to Washington. As we sat in the garden, talking, I told her about my search and my feeling that the "Old Testament" offered less to the person facing death than the "New," with its personification of God, its cross, and its dramatic resurrection. She said she would ask her father, Rabbi Louis Finkelstein, to write to me. I was delighted. I would be enlightened by one of the most renowned of Jewish scholars, the distinguished rabbi who had headed the Jewish Theological Seminary of America.

Handy kept her word. Her father's letter arrived at the end of 1979. Louis Finkelstein wrote that all authorities who were and are in the tradition have held that immortality of the soul is a basic dogma and that our stay here on earth is merely a prelude to a blessed and happy life. The reason that the biblical prophets avoided speaking of human mortality and resurrection of the dead is that, like most primitive men and women, the surrounding peoples of their time worshiped the dead. Since this was considered idolatry, they were hesitant to refer to the dead as still being alive. After the exile, this danger became remote, and thus leaders felt free to speak of human immortality.

Both in his letter to me and in a copy of one he enclosed to his granddaughter, Rabbi Finkelstein argued that there was no way of demonstrating such a doctrine in the scientific laboratory, but it was difficult for him to understand how a belief that is so widespread and makes so much sense of the riddle of human existence can be rejected. Death could not be very far off for him (indeed, he lived over a decade more), but it was nothing to be worried about because it would be like going from one room to another, only that in that second room, there are no troubles, no pains, no sickness, only joy and the opportunity to study.

Rabbi Finkelstein concluded that he had known many skeptics, but most had their belief hidden away somewhere in the back of their mind. Justice Felix Frankfurter, for instance, earnestly asked that the Kaddish be said when he died, and it was done. Well, I, too, want the Kaddish, the great mourner's prayer that does not mention death, said when I die; I want to be part of the continuity of the generations and of a great tradition. I, too, know I have some sort of belief—the psalmist's "rock" of the heart—hidden away at the back of my mind.

But it seemed to me that the rabbi was asking me to accept a great deal on faith—that death would be like going from one room to another, for example—simply because so many people smarter than I had done so. He didn't mention that other people smarter than I had not done so. I was disappointed in our correspondence.

Some twenty years later, I took a new look at this correspondence and its relation to my survivorship search for meaning with Daniel Zemel, Temple Micah's rabbi since 1983. In his typically uncritical fashion, Danny Zemel (as he is known to all) suggested that I not be so disappointed in Louis Finkelstein's attempt to enlighten me. I should realize, he said, that Finkelstein, like all of us, was the product of his time—which was more that of nineteenth-century Eastern Europe than late-twentieth-century Washington. For example, in his generation, it was enough—as Zemel's rabbinical school teacher had advised—to tell a congregant in personal trouble to "light the Shabbous candles." Defining spirituality as "the moment right now," he explained that nowadays, the act of lighting candles itself won't help anyone; you have to provide a context for it, so that it can become a spiritual connection to a bigger, grand picture—or it won't make sense.

As part of a national "Synagogue 2000" program, Temple Micah, under Rabbi Zemel's vigorous leadership, has been very much a part of the current effort in many faiths to make traditional religion more relevant to modern life (thawing the sitting-in-pews-staring-straight-ahead-being-lectured-to image of what an Episcopal friend calls "The Frozen People," linking hands or even hugging after services, and involving congregants in ways that would have confounded our grandparents). We were trying to help our rabbi turn around the assumption he quoted from a newspaper "personals" column wherein an AYJM (attractive young Jewish male) encapsulated his search for an AYJF (attractive young Jewish female) as someone who was, like himself, "spiritual, not religious." To find ways in which we could be both, I had participated in retreats and seminars and participatory "healing" services in which we congregants, usually against the background of beautiful music, had tried to tap into the wisdom of our religion, to find a more personal connection to God, stronger links to each other, and a more meaningful approach to our place in the sun.

Rather than putting me off, Rabbi Zemel continued, Louis Finkelstein had tried to give me what he knew. But times move on; change occurs; generations perceive differently; as I knew, the religious balance between the rational and the spiritual had begun to tip more toward the spiritual—toward concern for human feelings, for finding a personal connection with the eternal. (Here I thought of people like Judie Blanchard of the

National Coalition for Cancer Survivorship [NCCS], who finds genuine spiritual connections spending a week, absolutely silent, meditating with California monks, or rowing on the serene early morning Potomac, or joining a "Year to Live" group to reprioritize and do what is important *now*.)

Telling me simply to have faith that someone would be waiting in the next room, continued this rabbi who is in the same generation as Louis Finkelstein's granddaughter, meant something to that renowned man, but "telling it to you in your illness without a total context for the statement was like giving you the keys to a motorcycle but never giving you a lesson on how to ride one."

And though he did not call it that, Zemel gave me a short lesson in how to ride my spiritual motorcycle as we considered the lyrical words of the 139th Psalm, which I had studied in the Lombardi Cancer Center group, "Nourishing Our Spirits." This psalm (paraphrased at the end of the long Day of Atonement prayer book we use each year) echoed the notion of an eternal "rock" of the heart elucidated for me by Martin Buber.

Acknowledging that the Lord knows us completely and that we "cannot flee from your presence," the psalmist writes that even at the "farthest limits of the sea," God's right hand shall hold us fast:

> If I say, "Surely the darkness shall cover me,
> and the light around me become night,"
> even the darkness is not dark to you;
> the night is as bright as the day,
> for darkness is as light to you. . . .
>
> How weighty to me are your thoughts, O God!
> How vast the sum of them
> I try to count them—they are more than the sand;
> I come to the end—I am still with you.

He loves these last words, said Rabbi Zemel, because they seem so modern, so rational. I agree; these words underline what Ecclesiastes had already taught me: don't search too hard; we cannot understand, or even try to count, the "vast sum" of

God's "weighty" thoughts. They lie beyond the horizon of our minds. Only in this mysterious realm is God's mind found. But at the end, "I am still with you."

I had a longer lesson in how to ride my spiritual motorcycle when I was given the chance to get to know the prophet Jonah and make him part of my survivorship life. When the task of giving my personal spin on the story of Jonah on Yom Kippur afternoon fell to my lot as a member of the Micah congregation, I thought that Job was my particular prophet, or more accurately, biblical persona. In this I had been encouraged by friends and family who often made me vaguely uncomfortable by complimenting me for such attributes as "courage" and forbearance. I appreciated their words, but they usually made me squirm because I know my impatient self too well to look to Job as a role model for dealing patiently with the ups and downs of cancer.

As I studied and read over a period of many months, I came to claim Jonah, not Job, for a role model. Here indeed is a feisty, assertive human being struggling through improbable trials while his soul, as he puts it, grew "faint within him." Certainly —whether on the boat or in the belly of the whale or, later, sitting under a gourd outside Nineveh—he is not where he wanted to be. But he tries to live his hours and days constructively, a human being with faults doing his best by his conscience, his community, and his God. He remains his own person—the quintessential survivor.

Look at Jonah, for example, in the boat he hires at Jaffa to take him to faraway Tarshish (instead of going, as had been commanded, to Nineveh to warn its people to change their ways or be destroyed). A great storm comes up, a mighty wind churns the sea, threatening to break up the ship. His comrade sailors cry out to each other; they cast the ship's wares overboard to lighten it.

And where is Jonah? Down below, in the innermost parts of the ship, lying down, fast asleep. He is, as many a modern therapist has told lesser mortals dealing with threatening situations, *in denial.* Like many of us survivors, he refuses to confront what is happening to him. The ship's captain, much like a good friend or doctor or spouse today, has to shake him awake, crying,

"What meanest that thou sleepest? Arise! Call to your God. Perhaps God will pay us mind and we will not perish." Dragged back to face reality, he recognizes and accepts his responsibility to take action.

He does not have to find a new oncologist or medical center. He has to identify who he is, and in one of the most touching parts of the story, Jonah experiences something that, again, is very familiar to me as a survivor: *an unexpected and heartwarming solidarity with his fellow sufferers.* The sailors are not members of a support group, to be sure, exchanging information and survival hints. But they show him that they know they are indeed in the same boat. They make a real effort to save him, rowing hard to return to the shore.

When they fail, they respond to Jonah's command to heave him into the seas. They want to save him so badly that they do this gradually—lowering him into the water first up to his knees and pulling him back up, then to his navel and pulling him back, and when all that does not work, they submerge him completely, and the sea's wrath ceases. *So an important survivor contradiction exists: though we survive by helping one another, at the same time it is every human being for himself—or herself.*

In the most famous "ain't necessarily so" part of this story, Jonah, cast into the deep, swallowed by the great fish, is imprisoned alone in the fish's belly for three days and three nights. Presumably without oxygen, gasping for breath, he despairs. Like many a survivor, he undergoes a sort of *intensification of the inner life.* One might say he is depressed, and with good reason. Though he has escaped the anger of the sea, he knows he is in the netherworld, with death near. Still, he displays his courage. He elects to fight; he will not give in.

Out of his anguish, he prays. Rather than complain, as many of us less clever survivors might, his Psalm of Thanksgiving demonstrates his gratitude to God, who had, as he put it, "brought up my life from the pit." In this prayer, Jonah does what I—among millions of other survivors—have done in tough spots. *He bargains with God.* Like us modern survivors—when we promise that we will be more obedient children or more loving spouses or more giving community workers if only we can get through this round of chemo treatment or that surgery—he bargains:

> But as for me, with a cheer of gratitude
> Will I bring offerings to thee
> What I have vowed I will fulfill
> For the salvation which is the Lord's.

And the Lord speaks to the great fish, and it vomits Jonah out upon the dry land.

In the second part of this remarkable story, Jonah is given what every survivor prays for—*a second chance.* He has changed as a result of his experiences. He is more mature, more in command; he rolls more with the punches. He goes on to Nineveh, still the place he does not want to be, in accordance with God's wishes.

But he is still Jonah, the strong core of him still present, and he grows angry when he finds God too quick to accept the repentance of the people of Nineveh; he sees this divine forgiveness as an indictment against Israel, and thus of himself. His anger would not surprise any survivor struggling to stay afloat. *Anger,* the psychologists tell us, can be a pretty effective mask for anxiety about the ups and down of what is happening (as can humor, quite a different emotion). He leaves Nineveh and builds himself a booth outside the city to give himself some shade and await the outcome.

The prophet/survivor is on an emotional seesaw. He rejoices when God gives him a gourd to protect him from sun and wind. He is sheltered and comfortable, glad at this sign of God's love. But soon God sends a worm to wither the gourd, and I know *how faint this new affliction* makes him and why he asks for death. Reacting to cancer's repeated onslaughts, I have felt that way myself; in the aftermath of my nasty little tongue cancer surgery a few years ago, I suggested to my husband half jokingly that he get Dr. Kevorkian's phone number.

Still, at the end, Jonah seems to accept what has happened both to Nineveh and to himself. He does not answer directly when God tries to tell him that his word, his loving kindness, and his forgiveness are for all humankind. But we can answer for him, seeing that he accepts what has befallen both Nineveh and himself. He has taken *control of his experience, integrated it into his life.* We assume, we hope, that he has gone on to other things, much like the rest of us lesser survivors.

My new friend Jonah reaffirmed and enhanced a notion that has helped enormously in my personal survivor's search for meaning. I first heard it posited by a psychologist working with seriously ill patients who had turned to the literature of the Holocaust to learn about life in the extremity of life-threatening illness. Referring to Terrence Des Pres's remarkable book *The Survivor: An Anatomy of Life in the Death Camps,* he drew several important analogies between the two lives. In both, for instance, the extreme situation is neither an event nor a crisis with a beginning, middle, or end, but simply a state of existence, and always with the knowledge that death may win.

This is true for many—both for "rookie" and "veteran" survivors—though the degree of hope we harbor increases as time passes. Still, the idea of comparing my situation with that of a Holocaust victim seemed a bit pretentious, at first. I had not, after all, been beaten with whips, worn ragged clothing torn by dogs, breathed air so foul from excremental assault that no bird flew overhead. My survivor experiences seemed trivial compared with these humiliating horrors.

I ordered the Des Pres book, and while I waited for its arrival, I reread psychiatrist Viktor E. Frankl's *Man's Search for Meaning,* a compelling account of his own Holocaust/survivor experiences. When it came, *The Survivor,* which compiles actual testimony of survivors of Russian as well as Nazi death camps, fiercely and movingly underlined what I had acknowledged rereading Frankl through my newly found survivors' glasses. Indeed, there were many significant parallels between the survivor and the camp experiences, not so much in the terrible damage done to the human body in both worlds—nothing could equal the naked vilification of the Holocaust—as in the intensification of the inner life of those trapped there (which Jonah, too, had experienced in the great fish's belly). And in the clues this provided to the art of survival.

For both, as for Jonah and his sailor colleagues tossed danger-
ously on choppy seas, lives lived in extremity are collective acts.
No one survives without help. Extremity deepens relationships,
intensifies social bonding. In the camps, human beings were
reduced to a single mass of bone-thin festering bodies with
shaved heads, clad in filthy rags. They depended on each other,
propping up comrades when they lagged, exhausted and bare-
footed in the snow, hiding each other from brutal guards, smug-
gling a little extra food to satisfy each other's hunger, finding
great joy in service to others, whether it be giving each other
gifts—a potato, a leaf, a piece of string—or advice as to how to find
a clerical job. From each other they asked not pity, nor senti-
mentality, but support and camaraderie.

In hanging-in places, too, whether they be Sloan-Kettering
waiting rooms, midwestern church basements, or Cancer Help
Program retreats, we more fortunate survivors ask each other
less for pity or sympathy for our mutilated bodies than for proof
of friendship and caring. We support and encourage each other,
exchanging information of new drugs and treatments, rather
than food.

But if we do not watch out for ourselves, who will? When his
fellow sailors who had tried to help him were forced to throw
him overboard to still the seas, Jonah knew the contradiction:
though we survive by helping one another, it is everyone for
him- or herself. The prisoners learned how to work for, or even
in, camp administration, how to curry favors from the authorities, realistically and without illusion.

A strong sense of selfhood, or personhood, helped. Esther
Milgrom, my lawyer friend Toby Levin's mother, tells how she
escaped from a long line of naked prisoners bound for the gas
chambers at Auschwitz. She sighted a pile of clothes near the
barracks and knew that she, a self-respecting human being,
should be wearing them; once clothed, she became lost in a
crowd of laborers. Later, free in the United States, she remembers keeping the little floor space that was hers spotless, a
dignified shiny clean.

Of all the wealth of advantages freedom affords us cancer survivors—including family, friends, and support groups—none is

more crucial than the fact that our caretakers are just that, *care-takers*, who want to help rather than hurt us. As survivor Arthur Frank, the Canadian medical sociologist, put it in *The Wounded Storyteller*, suffering, the pain that isolates itself in conscious-ness, has its cry attended to, while the cry from the camp is left, stifled, "in its own uselessness." The SS guards took pleasure in telling Dachau inmates that they had no chance of coming out alive, and after the war the world would not believe what had happened. Our doctors, nurses, and counselors take pleasure and satisfaction, some with more success than others, in encourag-ing us to hope and to survive.

Less dramatically, we survivors learn the hard way how to deal with doctors and other caretakers who influence our lives. We learn firmly to distance ourselves from people whom we upset or who upset us. We learn to undertake only those tasks we can do realistically and to try to keep ourselves attractively groomed. I have not forgotten the memorial service for early breast cancer activist Rose Kushner, held at the National Institutes of Health, where speakers hailed not only her feisty advocacy and her net-working and legislative accomplishments but the snappy, fash-ionable way she dressed. No pitiable cancer patient, she.

Viktor Frankl tells how a wise senior block warden asked him to address his fellow prisoners at the end of a bad day in the camps. A semistarved prisoner had broken into a store to steal a few pounds of potatoes. Other prisoners had recognized the culprit, and the authorities ordered that the guilty man be given up. "Naturally, the 2,500 men preferred to starve."

Though cold and hungry, psychiatrist Frankl recognized an opportunity to encourage his comrades, lying about him, wan and exhausted on the earthen hut floor. Even in the sixth winter of the Second World War, he pointed out, their situation was not the most terrible they could imagine. After all, their bones were intact; they were still alive. They had reason to hope that health, family, fortune, happiness, professional careers would be restored.

No man, Frankl continued, knew what the future would bring. Though there was still no typhus in the camp, he estimated his own chances of surviving at about one in twenty. Still, he had no intention of losing hope, of giving up. Something might open up, the luck of attachment, for example, to a special group with good working conditions.

Turning to the past, the psychiatrist argued that no power on earth could take away what they had experienced, all they had suffered; even their seemingly hopeless struggle had dignity and meaning. Whatever they had gone through could be an asset in the future. He quoted Nietzsche: "That which does not kill me, makes me stronger." Those with any religious faith, he said, could understand that their sacrifice could have a meaning. And he told the miserable, pitiful friends around him about the man who made a pact with Heaven that his suffering should save the human being he loved the most from a painful end.

Jonah, again. And the rest of us survivors, who bargain with God and know that someone looking down on us, a God, a friend, a husband or wife (in Jonah's case, surely, God), will be disappointed if we do not know how to die, suffering proudly.

They were still alive, their bones intact. No intention of losing hope, something might open up. To die suffering proudly. Even in the most abnormal of lives in extremity, the way in which you deal with fate, the attitude you assume, gives deeper meaning to the days you have. Those who can step toward this deeper meaning and perform the acts of life accordingly often have the best chance for survival—either in the death camp or in the survivorship life.

Having a sense of humor, as many have noted, offers a definite advantage. Recognizing that humor offers the ability to rise above a situation, if only briefly, and thus is one of the soul's weapons in the fight for self-preservation, Viktor Frankl suggested to a surgeon friend that they tell each other an amusing story every day. In the same way, politician Hubert Humphrey stalked the Sloan-Kettering corridors in his bathrobe in the late 1970s, joshing and encouraging fellow patients, telling jokes. And twenty years later, non-Hodgkin's lymphoma (and bone marrow transplant) survivor Nancy Roth tickled hundreds attending NCCS's Tenth Annual Assembly in Albuquerque by presenting us with large improbable buttons declaring "Cancer

Sucks." (When he arrived and saw us wearing them, National Cancer Institute director Dr. Richard Klausner said he knew he was in the right place.)

Indeed, those who can find a kind of negative happiness in their situation have an advantage, too. They can say, with Dr. Frankl, that things are not as terrible as one would imagine, that they could be worse. They can find joy in an intricate flowering tree branch, or rainbow sunset, or small child's companionship. They can delight in working rhythmically and skillfully with a squad to build a wall in the freezing cold, or writing well, even isolated in a cancer transplant sickbed. They can, and do, believe something—deliverance from the Holocaust, a cure for cancer—will turn up.

Still, entering an unreal, provisional existence from which there is no set release date, human beings can be shocked to the point of collapse. In his afterword to *The Reawakening*, Primo Levi, another important and gifted witness to the Holocaust, pointed out that the total humiliation and demoralization prisoners suffered led many to "spiritual shipwreck." Terrorized, mourning, lacking information about what to do or how to act, they could lose their desire to fight for life. Lost in the poisoned nightmare of the Holocaust, the "walking dead" died before they were able to shake off their shock, wake to their predicament, and strike back. Lost in the perceived poisoned nightmare of treatment, cancer survivors can also give up before their time. In the clinics, you can always tell those few sad "shades," as a friend of mine called them, who have given up. Now, with more reason to hope, there are fewer and fewer "shade" folk and more cautiously optimistic ones. Hallelujah!

Those who survive can build a wall of apathy around themselves, denying that what is all about them is really happening. This has its own dangers: though apathy may keep despair at a distance, it can result in disregard for the environment, so that neither prisoner nor survivor strives to adapt to it. Fortunately in both worlds, many have emerged from apathy to struggle as best they can, refusing to see, even to consider, themselves "victims."

Survivors renew their stubborn will each morning, not always so much through what Terrence Des Pres calls "some

secret fortitude of the heart," but through the physical act of getting up, either from a few hours' sleep in a death camp or from a
troubled sickbed. The pain may be sharp, the misery deep, but
the commitment to another day must be made. In fact, the function of intelligence in extremity seems not so much to judge
your statistical chances as to make the most of the opportunity
of getting through each day. An Auschwitz survivor reported
that the sores on his feet opened as he climbed down and put on
his shoes each morning; he knew a new day had begun. Similarly, I have often felt, putting my luckier feet into my slippers
after a bad night, recommitted to another lucky stretch of
existence.

Finally, and this blew my mind when I first came upon it, there
was in the death camps, as Elie Wiesel has put it, "a veritable
passion to testify." The Holocaust produced an endless scream,
which in time was heard in the voices of an unusual number of
literate witnesses. Men and women knew they had to survive to
leave a trace, to tell people how they lived and died; they had to
survive to make the deathly silence speak, to erect a memorial
to millions of bodies burned in the gas chambers.

Des Pres reports that at Treblinka the inmates prepared to
destroy the camp so as to allow at least one man or woman to
live to tell the tale; forty survived. Two men, Michael Berg and
Alexander Donat, accidentally switched places in a death
brigade. Berg wrote *The Holocaust Kingdom* in Donat's name.
In *The Reawakening,* chemist Primo Levi asserts that he would
probably never have written anything had it not been for the
experience of the camp and the long journey home to Italy: "I did
not have to struggle with laziness, problems of style seemed
ridiculous to me, and miraculously I found the time to write. . . .
It seemed as if those books were all there, ready in my head, and
I had only to let them come out and pour onto paper."

The analogy to the survivor experience struck me forcibly.
"Death is compounded by oblivion," Des Pres observed, "and
the foundation of humanness—faith in continuity—is endan-
gered." Why else do so many of us survivors tell our stories
through articles, books, TV shows, and, now, on the Internet?

Why else did Barbara Saltzman, after her son David's death from a tumor that invaded his lungs in the 1990s, travel the country perpetuating the message of his book *The Jester Has Lost His Jingle,* about a jester who saves the world by making a young cancer survivor laugh?

In support groups, clinic waiting rooms, hospital corridors, over the telephone after I published a newspaper piece, I have met men and women who write, or want to write, about their experiences. Unlike the death camp survivors, they cannot with certainty hope that by so doing they will prevent a future repetition of their sufferings; they cannot cry "Never Again!" But like those other survivors, they can show that they were there and that what happened to them mattered. They can show their compassion for those who did not make it and their loyalty. They can try to help others by leaving them hints as to how to survive.

For Primo Levi, the brief and tragic camp experience had been overlaid with a much longer and complex experience as a writer-witness. In its totality, this past made him "richer and surer." Like a fellow deportee, who described the camp as her "university," he felt that "by living and then writing about and pondering about those events, I have learned many things about man and about the world." But Levi hastened to add that he remained acutely aware that only a tiny 5 percent of the Italian deportees returned, and he attributed his unharmed survival chiefly to good luck—with his training as a mountaineer and chemist playing only a small role. Perhaps, he mused, he was helped, too, by his never flagging interest in the human spirit, and the will "not only to survive (which was common to many) but with the precise purpose of recounting the things we had witnessed and endured."

I, too, chiefly credit good luck and the increased power of modern medicine for my longer ongoing survivorship experience. I, too, feel this unwanted experience, even in its darkest days, has made me and an increasing number of my fellow survivors richer and surer. I, too, wonder if I have been helped not only by my will to survive but by recounting the things I have witnessed and endured, and possibly, by helping others in similar straits.

I, too, have been helped by my never flagging interest in the resilience of the human spirit. This has deepened as I have seen some of my colleagues helping others voluntarily, unselfishly, others simply developing their talent for life, their ability to rely on the power of life itself. And it has swelled as I have watched them, like those who have preceded them, standing firm, learning, acknowledging the centrality of death, yet choosing life and seeking a high quality in that life; taking their stand right on the line, staying there, hanging in, even when their will to go on may seem illogical. In this way, the ordeal of the survivor becomes an experience of growth and self-realization.

The Cancer Survivors' Bill of Rights

A new population lives among us today—a new minority of 8 million people with a history of cancer. Four million of these Americans have lived with their diagnoses for five years or more.

You see these modern survivors in offices and in factories, on bicycles and cruise ships, on tennis courts, beaches, and bowling alleys. You see them in all ages, shapes, sizes, and colors. Usually they are unremarkable in appearance, sometimes they are remarkable for the way they have learned to live with disabilities resulting from cancer or its treatment.

Modern medical advances have returned over half of the nation's cancer patients of all ages to a normal lifespan. But the larger society has not always kept pace in helping make this lifespan truly "normal." At least, it has felt awkward in dealing with this fledgling group; at most, it has failed fully to accept survivors as functioning members.

The American Cancer Society presents this Survivors' Bill of Rights to call public attention to survivor needs, to enhance cancer care, and to bring greater satisfaction to cancer survivors, as well as to their physicians, employers, families, and friends:

The Cancer Survivors' Bill of Rights was initially written by Natalie Davis Spingarn for the American Cancer Society in 1988 and is now available from the National Coalition for Cancer Survivorship, 1010 Wayne Avenue, Suite 505, Silver Spring, MD 20910.

1. Survivors have the right to assurance of lifelong medical care, as needed. The physicians and other professionals involved in their care should continue their constant efforts to be:
   —sensitive to the cancer survivors' lifestyle choices and their need for self-esteem and dignity;
   —careful, no matter how long their patients have survived, to take symptoms seriously, and not dismiss aches and pains, for fear of recurrence is a normal part of survivorship;
   —informative and open, providing survivors with as much or as little candid medical information as they wish, and encouraging their informed participation in their own care;
   —knowledgeable about counseling resources, and willing to refer survivors and their families as appropriate for emotional support and therapy which will improve the quality of individual lives.

2. In their personal lives, survivors, like other Americans, have the right to the pursuit of happiness. This means they have the right:
   —to talk with their families and friends about their cancer experience if they wish, but to refuse to discuss it if that is their choice, and not to be expected to be more upbeat or less blue than anyone else;
   —to be free of the stigma of cancer as a "dread disease" in all social relations;
   —to be free of blame for having gotten the disease and of guilt for having survived it.

3. In the work place, survivors have the right to equal job opportunities. This means they have the right:
   —to aspire to jobs wo rthy of their skills, and for which they are trained and experienced, and thus not to have to accept jobs they would not have considered before the cancer experience;
   —to be hired, promoted, and accepted on return to work, according to their individual abilities and qualifications, and not according to "cancer" or "disability" stereotypes;
   —to privacy about their medical histories.

4. Since health insurance coverage is an overriding survivorship concern, every effort should be made to assure all survivors adequate health insurance, whether public or private. This means:
   —for employers, that survivors have the right to be included in group health coverage, which is usually less expensive, provides better benefits, and covers the employees regardless of health history;
   —for physicians, counselors, and other professionals concerned, that they keep themselves and their survivor-clients informed and up-to-date on available group or individual health policy options, noting, for example, what major expenses like hospital costs and medical tests outside the hospital are covered and what amount must be paid before coverage (deductible);
   —for social policy makers, both in government and in the private sector, that they seek to broaden insurance programs like Medicare to include diagnostic procedures and treatment which help prevent recurrence and ease survivor anxiety and pain.

❧ *Notes*

A wealth of information accumulated over many years, enriched by more than fifty recently taped interviews, went into the writing of this book. To make this material accessible to the reader yet at the same time avoid ponderous citations throughout the text, I've combined references to published sources with explanatory notes and suggestions for further reading, indexed by page.

Preface

ix   There are several "good cancer books" available. For personal tales, see Betty Rollin, *First, You Cry* (New York: Signet, 1976), and Gilda Radner, *It's Always Something* (New York: Simon and Schuster, 1989). For dispassionate books on special cures, see Barrie R. Cassileth, *The Alternative Medicine Handbook: The Complete Reference Guide to Alternative and Complementary Therapies* (New York: W. W. Norton, 1998), and Michael Lerner, *Choices in Healing: Integrating the Best of Conventional and Complementary Approaches to Cancer* (Cambridge: MIT Press, 1996). For material on different aspects of survivorship, see Marion Morra and Eve Potts, *Choices: Realistic Alternatives in Cancer Treatment* (New York: Avon, 1980) and *Triumph: Getting Back to Normal When You Have Cancer* (New York: Avon, 1990); see also Sidney J. Winawer et al., *Cancer Free* (New York: Simon and Schuster, 1995).

x   Natalie Davis Spingarn, "Breast Cancer: New Choices," *Washington Post*, Outlook section, December 22, 1974, B1; see also "My Mind vs. My Cancer," September 13, 1981, C1, and other articles on breast cancer published in the *Post* between 1974 and 1981.

See also Natalie Davis Spingarn, *Hanging in There: Living Well on Borrowed Time* (Briarcliff Manor, N.Y.: Stein and Day, 1982). The paperback edition appeared in 1984.

Anatole Broyard, "Good Books about Being Sick," *New York Times Book Review*, April 1, 1980, 1, 28–29.

1   *Hanging In There*

1   General information about cancer risk and available treatments, current research, and patient resources can be obtained from the National Cancer Institute (1-800-4-CANCER, 9:00 A.M. to 4:30 P.M., Monday–Friday) and from the American Cancer Society (1-800-227-2345, 24 hours a day, 7 days a week). The *Cancer Risk Report*, published annually by the American Cancer Society, is also a good resource.

For statistics and trends, see also *Cancer Facts and Figures*, a widely used compendium published annually by the American Cancer Society. In addition, the National Cancer Institute *Fact Book*, which contains data from the Surveillance, Epidemiology, and End Results (SEER) program, is published annually by the National Institutes of Health, U.S. Department of Health and Human Services.

For the upbeat "report card" published by the American Cancer Society, National Cancer Institute, and Centers for Disease Control and Prevention, see Phyllis A. Wingo et al., "Cancer Incidence and Mortality, 1973–1995: A Report Card for the U.S.," *Cancer* 82, no. 6 (March 15, 1998): 1197–1207. The 1999 report (reports are published annually), which appeared in the April issue of the *Journal of the National Cancer Institute*, indicated a continuation of the same general trends.

8   Center for Attitudinal Healing, *There Is a Rainbow behind Every Dark Cloud* (Tiburon, Calif., 1978).

9   See Stewart Alsop, *Stay of Execution* (New York: Harper & Row, 1973).

Wendy Schlessel Harpham, *When a Parent Has Cancer: A Guide to Caring for Your Children*, including a special book for children, *Becky and the Worry Cup* (New York: HarperCollins, 1997). Also by Harpham, see *Diagnosis Cancer: Your Guide through the First Few Months* (New York: W. W. Norton, 1992) and *After Cancer: A Guide to Your New Life* (New York: W. W. Norton, 1994).

2   *The Bad News*

12   George V. Coelho, with David A. Hamburg and John E. Adams, eds., *Coping and Adaptation* (New York: Basic Books, 1974). See also David A. Hamburg and John E. Adams, "A Perspective on Coping Behavior," *Archives of General Psychiatry* 17 (September 1967): 277–84, and Julia H. Rowland, "Intrapersonal Resources: Coping," in *The Handbook of Psychooncology*, ed. Jimmie C. Holland and Julia H. Rowland (New York: Oxford University Press, 1989), 44–57.

14   George Crile Jr., *What Women Should Know about the Breast Cancer Controversy* (New York: Pocket Books, 1974).

15   For information concerning statements put out by the National Institutes of Health Consensus Panels, contact the Office of Medical Applications of Research, National Institutes of Health, Bethesda, Maryland, (301) 496-1144.

20   For the article on Washington's "top doctors" (with mention of Dr. Katherine Alley), see Carol Stevens, "Good Medicine," *Washingtonian* (November 1993): 91–95, 98.

22   Monica Morrow, with Cathy Bucci and Alfred Rademaker, "Medical Con-
     traindications Are Not a Major Factor in the Underutilization of Breast
     Conserving Therapy," *Journal of the American College of Surgeons* 185,
     no. 9 (March 1998): 269.
          Material regarding types of breast augmentations was provided by the
     Plastic Surgery Information Service of the American Society of Plastic and
     Reconstructive Surgeons, Arlington Heights, Illinois.
25   See Sandra Day O'Connor, "Surviving Cancer: A Private Person's Public
     Tale," *Washington Post*, Health section, November 8, 1994, 7.

3   *Talking and Hoping*

28   "Consider the Source: Respondents Rate 12 Health Information Sources,"
     The Patient's Network (TPN) 2, no. 1 (Summer 1997): 3–5. This quarterly
     newsletter is published by the International Alliance of Patients' Organiza-
     tions (IAPO), which advocates on behalf of patients in international health
     care policy arenas. For information, write to Joanne Nelson, Wellness Inter-
     action Network, 10430 Oklahoma Avenue, Chatsworth, CA 91311.
29   Elisabeth Kübler-Ross, *On Death and Dying* (New York: Macmillan, 1969).
30   On the "policy turn-about," see Dennis H. Novack et al., "Changes in
     Physicians' Attitudes toward Telling the Cancer Patient," *Journal of the
     American Medical Association* 241, no. 9 (March 2, 1979): 897–900. For
     results of the Philadelphia study, see Edward Gottheil et al., "Awareness
     and Disengagement in Cancer Patients," *American Journal of Psychiatry*
     136, no. 5 (May 1979): 632–36.
          For more on patient-doctor communications, see Ernest Rosenbaum
     and Isadora Rosenbaum, "Achieving Open Communication with Cancer
     Patients through Audio and Videotapes," *Journal of Psychosocial Oncol-
     ogy* 4, no. 4 (Winter 1986): 91–105. Also see Natalie Davis Spingarn and
     Nancy H. Chasen, "Working with Your Doctor and Hospital System:
     Becoming a Wise Consumer," in *A Cancer Survivor's Almanac*, ed. Bar-
     bara Hoffman (Minneapolis: Chronimed, 1996), 31–60.
34   *Patients and Doctors: Communication Is a Two-Way Street*, written by
     Natalie Davis Spingarn, produced by Ricki Green and Jill Clevinger, with
     support from the American Cancer Society and the Picker Foundation.
     Running time 22 minutes. (The film is now out of circulation.)
36   For the effects of poor patient-doctor communications on patients' health,
     see Sherrie Kaplan, Sheldon Greenfield, and J. E. Ware Jr., "Implications of
     Doctor-Patient Relationships for Patients' Health Outcomes," in *Commu-
     nicating with Patients in Medical Practice*, ed. M. Stewart and D. L. Roter
     (Newbury Park, Calif.: Sage, 1989), 228–45. See also Sheldon Greenfield et
     al., "Expanding Patient Involvement in Care: Effects on Patient Out-
     comes," *Annals of Internal Medicine* 102, no. 4 (1985): 520–28.
38   For the *Times* article featuring the Dalai Lama, see Nadine Brozan, "Spiri-
     tuality and Medicine," *New York Times*, Metro section, July 18, 1998.
          Information about courses teaching communications skills is based on
     personal communication with Barbara Barzansky, director of Medical

School Services, American Medical Association, October 10, 1997. Statistics are from the Liaison Committee on Medical Education's Annual Medical School Questionnaire, 1996–97.

For more on communications in the era of managed care, see David Mechanic and Mark Schlesinger, "The Impact of Managed Care on Patients' Trust in Medical Care and Their Physicians: The Patient-Physician Relationship," *Journal of the American Medical Association* 275, no. 21 (June 5, 1996): 1693–95.

Emily Dickinson, "Hope is the thing with feathers," in *The Complete Poems of Emily Dickinson,* ed. Thomas H. Johnson (Boston: Little, Brown, 1951).

39   Natalie Davis Spingarn, "How Am I?" *Parade,* October 9, 1983, 14–15. For more on coping, see Avery D. Weisman, *Coping with Cancer* (New York: McGraw-Hill, 1979).

40   Arnold A. Hutschnecker, *Hope: The Dynamics of Self-Fulfillment* (New York: G. P. Putnam's Sons, 1981).

41   For an older review of the literature on psychological states and bodily disease, including the study of "hopeless" patients, see Jerome D. Frank, "Psychotherapy of Bodily Disease: An Overview," *Psychotherapy and Psychosomatics* 26, no. 4 (1975): 192–202. See also the more recent volume by Drs. Jerome P. Frank and Julia B. Frank, *Persuasion and Healing: A Comparative Study of Psychotherapy,* 3d ed. (Baltimore: Johns Hopkins University Press, 1993).

Elizabeth J. Clark, *Words That Heal, Words That Harm* and also *You Have the Right to Be Hopeful* (Silver Spring, Md.: National Coalition for Cancer Survivorship, 1995).

42   C. R. Snyder, *The Psychology of Hope* (New York: Free Press, 1994).

43   Mary L. Nowotny, "Assessment of Hope in Patients with Cancer: Development of An Instrument," *Oncology Nursing Forum* 16, no. 1 (1989): 57–61. See also "Every Tomorrow, a Vision of Hope," *Journal of Psychosocial Oncology* 9, no. 3 (1991): 117–25.

For more about the UCLA study, see Natalie Davis Spingarn, "Your Illusions May Be Good for You," *Parade,* March 10, 1985, 12. The article cited findings by Shelly E. Taylor, R. R. Lichtman, and J. V. Wood, "Attributions, Beliefs about Control, and Adjustment to Breast Cancer," *Journal of Personality and Social Psychology* 46, no. 3 (1984): 489–502. See also Shelly E. Taylor, *Positive Illusions: Creative Self-Deception and the Healthy Mind* (New York: Basic Books, 1989).

44   For the Dana-Farber study on misplaced hope, see Jane Weeks et al., "Relationship between Cancer Patients' Predictions of Prognosis and Their Treatment Preferences," *Journal of the American Medical Association* 279, no. 21 (June 3, 1998): 1709–14. Also see the accompanying JAMA editorial by Thomas J. Smith, "Telling the Truth about Cancer." For a report on this study, see Susan Gilbert, "For Cancer Patients, Hope Can Add to Pain," *New York Times,* Health section, June 9, 1998, C7. See also Janet H. Greenhut, "Living without Hope," *Second Opinion* 21, no. 1 (July 1995): 27–33.

4 *Being Sick*

49 Robert Lipsyte, *In the Country of Illness* (New York: Knopf, 1998).

52 Norman Cousins, *Anatomy of an Illness* (New York: W. W. Norton, 1979).

57 Fitzhugh Mullan, "Pain: Just Say No," *Networker* 8, no. 1 (Spring 1994): 2. National Coalition for Cancer Survivorship.

58 Kathleen Foley, "Pain Relief into Practice: Rhetoric without Reform," *Journal of Clinical Oncology* 13, no. 9 (September 1995): 2149–51. See also "Kill the Pain, Not the Patient," *Data Base,* a publication of the Dana Alliance for Brain Initiatives, November 25, 1996, and "Supportive Care and Quality of Life," in *Cancer: Principles and Practice of Oncology,* 5th ed., ed. Vincent T. DeVita et al. (Philadelphia: Lippincott-Raven, 1997), 2807–41.

59 For coverage of the Betsy Lehman story, including the Yale Cancer Center's survey of changes in chemotherapy safety procedures, see reporting by Richard Knox in the *Boston Globe* during 1995 and 1996, especially "Chemotherapy Deaths Spur Safer Methods," December 23, 1996, B1. See also Natalie Davis Spingarn, "Doctors Can Prevent Errors Just by Listening," letter to the editor of the *New York Times,* published July 25, 1995.

60 The author's list of suggestions for dealing with hospital life was printed in *A Cancer Survivor's Almanac,* ed. Barbara Hoffman (Minneapolis: Chronimed, 1996), 49.

5 *A New Subculture*

65 Natalie Davis Spingarn, "The New Breed of Survivors," *Washington Post,* Health section, April 10, 1985, 3.

66 For more on the acute, extended, and permanent stages of treatment, see Fitzhugh Mullan, "Seasons of Survival: Reflections of a Physician with Cancer," *New England Journal of Medicine* 313 (July 25, 1985): 270–73. Also, Natalie Davis Spingarn, "Letter to the Editor," *New England Journal of Medicine* 314, no. 3 (January 16, 1986): 188.

68 Arthur W. Frank, *At the Will of the Body* (Boston: Houghton Mifflin, 1991).

69 For stories of "gallant young survivors," see Beth Miller, "Sharing Her Life, Her Fight, Her Death," *Wilmington News Journal,* July 15, 1997, D1–D2, and also Karen Avenoso, "In a Place Hard to Reach," *Boston Globe,* July 23, 1997, D1, D4–D5.

 For information about meetings of the President's Cancer Panel, or to request transcripts, write to the President's Cancer Panel, National Cancer Institute, 31 Center Drive, Building 31, Bethesda, MD 20892-2743, or fax to (301) 402-1508.

71 See "Many-Faceted Program Helps Map 'Other Bank,'" *Networker* 3, no. 4 (Fall 1989): 1, 3–4. National Coalition for Cancer Survivorship.

73 Wenda Wardell Morrone, "Bridges," *Glamour* (September 1997): 180.

 For the poem "Ode to my Cancer-Ridden Body," see Barbara Boggs Sigmund, *An Unfinished Life* (Princeton, N.J.: Princeton University Press, 1990), 2–3.

77 For information about Life After Cancer Care, call the M. D. Anderson Information line at 1-800-392-1611, option 3.

Natalie Davis Spingarn, "NCI Devotes Tiny Percent of Budget Survivorship Research, but Plans to Move Forward," *Networker* 2, no. 3 (Summer 1988): 3–4. National Coalition for Cancer Survivorship.

6   Tools and Crutches

81   The National Coalition for Cancer Survivorship is a good resource for regional support group information. For general information, call (877) 622-7937 or write to NCCS, 1010 Wayne Avenue, Silver Spring, MD 20910. On the Internet, see www.cansearch.org.

87   Cancer Care teleconferences are free and open to the public. For information or to register, call 1-800-813-HOPE, or write to Cancer Care, Inc., 1180 Avenue of the Americas, New York, NY 10036.

88   *Privacy and American Business*, a newsletter published by the Center for Social and Legal Research, is a good source for health confidentiality and privacy issues. Contact them at Two University Plaza, Suite 414, Hackensack, NJ 07601; (201) 996-1154 or fax (201) 996-1883.

91   Stephen P. Hersh, *Beyond Miracles: Living with Cancer* (Lincolnwood, Ill.: Contemporary Books, 1998).

92   Vivian Iacovino and Kenneth Reesor, "Literature on Interventions to Address Cancer Patients' Psychosocial Needs: What Does It Tell Us?" *Journal of Psychosocial Oncology* 15, no. 2 (1997): 47–71.

For practical information about professional care providers, including how to find them, what to expect, and how they can help you, see Diane Blum, "The Healthcare Team: Working Together for Your Benefit," in *A Cancer Survivor's Almanac*, ed. Barbara Hoffman (Minneapolis: Chronimed, 1996), 61–71.

7   Complementary and Alternative Therapies

98   Yoga meditations from Izumi Shikibu, "Watching the Moon," trans. Jane Hirshfield with Mariko Aratani, in *The Enlightened Heart: An Anthology of Sacred Poetry*, ed. Stephen Mitchell (New York: Harper & Row, 1989), 40. For chants, including "The Five Remembrances," see *Plum Village Chanting Book*, ed. Thich Nhat Han (Berkeley, Calif.: Parallax Press, 1998).

105   Lawrence LeShan, *You Can Fight for Your Life* (New York: M. Evans, 1977).

106   Evan Handler, *Time On Fire* (New York: Owl Books, 1996).

107   Brallier tapes, including "Suggestions for Restful Sleep" and "Suggestions for General Relaxation," can be obtained from the Stress and Health Management Center, (202) 543-4945 or 1-888-553-4010. On the Internet, access www.healthhelpers.com.

108   Stephen P. Hersh, *Beyond Miracles: Living with Cancer*. See above, chapter 6.

109   For the report on the Prince of Wales, see "Prince Pioneers Alternative Options," *London Daily Telegraph*, October 21, 1997, 13.

David M. Eisenberg et al., "Trends in Alternative Medicine Use in the United States, 1990–1997," *Journal of the American Medical Association* 280, no. 18 (November 11, 1998): 1569–75. Also see the earlier study by David M. Eisenberg et al., "Unconventional Medicine in the United

States," *New England Journal of Medicine* 328 (January 28, 1995): 246–52.

110 George Ritzer, *The McDonaldization of Society: An Investigation into the Changing Character of Contemporary Social Life* (Newbury Park, Calif.: Sage Books/Pine Forge Press, 1993).

111 David Spiegel, *Living beyond Limits* (New York: Times Books, 1993); also David Spiegel et al., "Effect of Psychosocial Treatment on Survival of Patients with Metastatic Breast Cancer," *Lancet* 2 (October 14, 1989): 888–91.

Also, Michael Lerner, *Choices in Healing*, and Barrie R. Cassileth, *The Alternative Medicine Handbook*. See above, preface.

114 Information about shark cartilage from Denis R. Miller et al., "Phase I/II Trial of the Safety and Efficacy of Shark Cartilage in the Treatment of Advanced Cancer," *Journal of Clinical Oncology* 16, no. 11 (November 1998): 3649–55.

116 Robert M. Sapolsky, *Why Zebras Don't Get Ulcers* (New York: W. H. Freeman, 1994).

117 D. H. Bovbjerg and H. B. Valdimarsdottir, "Psychoneuroimmunology: Implications for Psychooncology," in *Textbook of Psycho-Oncology*, ed. Jimmie Holland et al. (New York: Oxford University Press, 1998), 125–34.

118 I. F. Fawzy et al., "Malignant Melanoma: Effects of Early Structured Psychiatric Intervention, Coping, and Affective State on Recurrence and Survival Six Years Later," *Archives of General Psychiatry* 50, no. 9 (September 1993): 681–89.

119 David Spiegel, "Psychological Distress and Disease Course for Women with Breast Cancer: One Answer, Many Questions," *Journal of the National Cancer Institute* 88, no. 10 (May 15, 1996): 629.

For more on the difficulties inherent in the scientific replication of the Siegel-Fawzy studies, see G. A. Gellert, R. M. Maxwell, and B. S. Siegel, "Survival of Breast Cancer Patients Receiving Adjunctive Psychosocial Support Therapy: A 10-Year Follow-Up Study," *Journal of Clinical Oncology* 11, no. 1 (January 1993): 66–69.

8 Significant Others

123 The "Funny Family" comes from Barbara Mathias, "Friends in Deed," *Washington Post*, January 2, 1996, C5. See also Cappy Capossela and Sheila Warnock, *Share the Care: How to Organize a Group to Care for Someone Who Is Seriously Ill* (New York: Fireside, 1995).

125 Marguerite S. Lederberg, "The Family of the Cancer Patient," in *Textbook of Psycho-Oncology*, ed. Jimmie Holland et al. (New York: Oxford University Press, 1998), 981–93.

126 Laura E. Nathan, "Coping with Uncertainty: Family Members' Adaptations during Cancer Remission," in *Clinical Sociological Perspectives on Illness and Loss: The Linkage of Theory and Practice*, ed. Elizabeth J. Clark et al. (Philadelphia: Charles Press, 1990), 219–33.

128   See Marisa C. Weiss and Ellen Weiss, *Living beyond Breast Cancer: A Survivor's Guide for When Treatment Ends and the Rest of Your Life Begins* (New York: Times Books, 1997). For Wendy Harpham's books, see above, chapter 1.

133   "Gravy," in Raymond Carver, *A New Path to the Waterfall* (New York: Atlantic Monthly Press, 1989), 118.

    The Sixth Biennial Symposium on Minorities, the Medically Underserved, and Cancer was held April 23–27, 1997, in Washington, D.C. Paper abstracts and information about other symposia can be obtained from the Intercultural Cancer Council, 1720 Dryden, Suite C, Houston, TX 77030; (713) 798-4617.

136   For general information on genetics and genetic counseling, contact the Alliance of Genetic Support Groups at 1-800-336-GENE, or 4301 Connecticut Avenue NW, Suite 404, Washington, DC 20008. *The Patient's Network* (see above, chapter 3) is another good resource; see the Spring 1997 issue, "Special Supplement: Human Genomics." Also, "What Can Our Genes Tell Us?" *Harvard Women's Health Watch* (July 1998), and Jerome Groopman, "Decoding Destiny," *New Yorker* (February 9, 1998): 42–47.

9   *The Media and the Message*

141   For 1998 breast cancer statistics, see the American Cancer Society, *Cancer Facts and Figures—1999*, available from the ACS at 1-800-ACS-2345.

142   "Icy Aid for Cancer Victims," *Newsweek* (September 17, 1979): 89.

143   The conference "Breakthrough! How News Influences Health Perception and Behavior" was held at the Cold Spring Harbor Laboratory, February 27–March 1, 1998. References in the text are from the author's personal communications with Victor Cohen, Kirsten Boyd Goldberg, and Barbara Rimer. To learn more about "Breakthrough," see "Conference Explores Hype and Hope in Communicating Science News," special edition of the *Cancer Letter* 24, no. 19 (May 15, 1998).

145   The National Health Council survey, conducted by Roper Starch Worldwide, was released in December 1997. Results were based on telephone interviews with a nationwide cross section of 2,256 adults in the United States. For an executive summary or for the full report, contact the National Health Council at 1730 M Street NW, Suite 500, Washington, DC 20036; (202) 785-3910.

146   For stories about patients seeking health information on the Internet, see Ken Mott, "Cancer and the Internet," *Surviving* (Winter 1997): 11, 14. Reprinted from *Newsweek* (August 19, 1996). Also, Katie Hafner, "The Doctor Is On," *Newsweek* (May 17, 1996): 78–79; Laura Johannes, "Medicine: Patients Delve into Databases to Second-Guess Doctors," *Wall Street Journal*, February 21, 1996, B1; and Mary Beth Franklin, "Researching Your Own Disease," *Washington Post*, Health section, August 4, 1998, 10, 12–13.

    On finding "credible and useful Web sites," see "Quality of Health Information on the Internet: Enabling Consumers to Tell Fact from Fraud," report available from the Health Improvement Institute, 5272 River Road, Suite 650, Bethesda, MD 20816; (301) 652-1250. Information is also posted on the institute's Web site at www.hii.org. See also Alejandro R. Jadad and Anna Gagliardi, "Rating Health Information on the Internet: Navigating to Knowledge or to Babel?" *Journal of the American Medical Association* 279, no. 8 (February 25, 1998): 611–14, and Brad Keoun, "Cancer Patients Find Quackery on the Web," *Journal of the National Cancer Institute* 88, no. 88 (September 18, 1996): 1263–65.

148 For information on NIH Consensus Statements, see above, chapter 2.

153 Number of calls following the October 1997 broadcast of the *Murphy Brown* show from the Susan G. Komen Breast Cancer Foundation, 5005 LBJ Freeway, Suite 250, Dallas, TX 75244; (972) 855-1600. For more information, see www.breastcancerinfo.com.

154 About the Ovarian Cancer National Alliance and its efforts to focus attention on ovarian cancer, see Letty Cottin Pogrebin, "Ovarian Cancer: Women Break the Silence," *Ms.* (March/April 1998): 34–36.

155 See Susan Sontag, *Illness as Metaphor* (New York: Doubleday Anchor, 1989). Also Arthur Frank, *At the Will of the Body* (Boston: Houghton Mifflin, 1991).

159 For my review of Bernie Siegel's book *Peace, Love, and Healing* (New York: Harper & Row, 1989), see "Self-Love and Healing Messages," *Washington Post*, September 26, 1989, 17. For his earlier book, see Bernie Siegel, *Love, Medicine, and Miracles* (New York: Harper & Row, 1986).

10   *Work*

160 Details of the Karuschkat story are from personal interviews with Jane Karuschkat, Barbara Hoffman, and others. See also Karuschkat, "Breast Cancer Cost Me My Job," *Ladies' Home Journal* (February 1998): 32, 46.

163 Studs Terkel, *Working* (New York: Pantheon, 1974).

For the Feldman studies, see *Work and Cancer Health Histories*, a series of reports by Frances Lomas Feldman distributed by the California Division of the American Cancer Society, San Francisco. Included in the series are "A Study of the Experiences of Recovered Patients" (May 1976); "A Study of the Experiences of Blue Collar Workers" (September 1978); and "Work Expectations and Experiences of Youth (Ages 13–23) with Cancer Histories" (July 1980).

167 Susan Scherr, "Benefits of Worksite Screening: Survivors Tell Their Stories," in *Cancer Screening and the Workplace: A Comprehensive Guide to Launching a Cancer Education, Prevention, and Screening Program in Your Company*, Industries' Coalition Against Cancer (ICAP), 1997. Available from PRR, Inc., 17 Prospect Street, Huntington, NY 11743.

168 See Barbara Hoffman, "Working It Out: Your Employment Rights," in *A Cancer Survivor's Almanac*, ed. Barbara Hoffman (Minneapolis: Chronimed, 1996).

170 For more on the Americans with Disabilities Act (ADA), see Barbara Hoffman, "One Way Up, One All the Way Down," *Networker* 4, no. 3 (Summer

1990): 9. National Coalition for Cancer Survivorship. Also, "Three Lessons from the Courtroom," *Networker* 12, no. 1 (Spring 1998): 3, 20.

173   The Amgen survey was conducted by CDB Research & Consulting, Inc., and published in the report *Cancer Discrimination in the Workplace: A National Assessment of Survivor Experiences* (Thousand Oaks, Calif.: Amgen, 1996). For a story about the Amgen survey, see Lauren Chambliss, "The Cancer Reality Gap," *Working Woman Magazine* (October 1996): 47–49, 68.

"Work! Thank God for the swing of it" from the poem by Angela Morgan, "Work: A Song of Triumph," *Bartlett's Quotations*, 13th ed. (Boston: Little, Brown, 1955), s.v. *work*.

11   *Money*

179   Statistics on cancer incidence and mortality can be found in the American Cancer Society "Report Card for the U.S." See above, chapter 1.

180   Nancy Breen, Larry G. Kessler, and Martin L. Brown, "Breast Cancer Control among the Underserved: An Overview," *Breast Cancer Research and Treatment* 40, no. 1 (1996): 105–15. See also Nancy Breen and Janis Barry Figueroa, "Stage of Breast and Cervical Cancer Diagnosis in Disadvantaged Neighborhoods: A Prevention Policy Perspective," *American Journal of Preventive Medicine* 12, no. 5 (1996): 319–25, and "Significance of Underclass Residence on the Stage of Breast or Cervical Cancer Diagnosis," *AEA Papers and Proceedings* 85, no. 2 (May 1995): 112–15.

Information about minorities and cancer is available from the Intercultural Cancer Council. See above, chapter 8.

181   Concerning the cost of care, see Bruce Fireman et al., "Cost of Care for Cancer in a Health Maintenance Organization," *Health Care Financing Review* 18, no. 4 (Summer 1997): 51–76. See also M. L. Brown and L. Fintor, "Cost Effectiveness of Breast Cancer Screening: Preliminary Results of a Systematic Review of the Literature," *Breast Cancer Research and Treatment* no. 25 (1993): 113–18.

182   American Association for Cancer Research (AACR) Fact Sheet, "Recent Progress and Future Opportunities in Breast Cancer Research," April 1997.

185   For the comparative study of women living in the San Francisco–Oakland and Seattle–Puget Sound areas, see Arnold L. Potosky et al., "Breast Cancer Survival and Treatment in Health Maintenance Organization and Fee-for-Service Settings," *Journal of the National Cancer Institute* 89, no. 22 (November 19, 1997): 1683–91.

186   U.S. Department of Commerce, Economics and Statistics Administration, "Health Insurance Coverage: 1997," Census Bureau Report P60-202 by Robert L. Bennefield, September 1998.

187   Myra Glajchen, "Psychosocial Consequences of Inadequate Health Insurance for Patients with Cancer," *Cancer Practice* 2, no. 2 (March/April 1994): 115–20. See also Myra Glajchen et al., "Psychosocial Impact of Insurance Coverage for People with Cancer" (paper delivered at the World Congress of Psycho-Oncology, New York, October 1996).

188   See Peter T. Kilborn, "Poor Workers Turning Down Employers' Health
      Benefits," *New York Times*, November 10, 1997, A24. Also "Unlearned,
      Unhealthy, and Mostly Uninsured," *New York Times*, August 5, 1997, A12.
         For the Michael Mulloy story, see Bob Herbert, "A Chance to Survive,"
      New York Times, July 4, 1997, A19.

190   State-by-state information about consumer rights to health insurance
      under the Health Insurance Portability and Accountability Act (the Kasse-
      baum-Kennedy law)—and under other insurance reform laws—is available
      from Georgetown University Institute for Health Care Research and Pol-
      icy, Washington, DC 20007. A useful guide is posted on the Internet at
      www.georgetown.edu/research/ihcrp/hipaa, and "What Cancer Survivors
      Need to Know about Health Insurance," a pamphlet prepared by Karen Pol-
      litz and Kimberley Calder (1993), is available from the NCCS.

191   Diana Sugg, "Activist Gaddy Announces That She Has Breast Cancer,"
      Baltimore Sun, April 22, 1998, 1B.

192   This definition of quality health care is from the National Academy of Sci-
      ence, Institute of Medicine. See *Medicare: A Strategy for Quality Assur-
      ance*, ed. K. N. Lohr (Washington, D.C.: National Academy Press, 1990).
         For statistics on variations in the quality of breast cancer care from
      state to state, see Dartmouth Medical School, Center for the Evaluative
      Clinical Sciences, *The Dartmouth Atlas of Health Care in the United
      States* (Chicago: American Hospital Publishing, 1996).

193   "Report Cards" from the National Committee for Quality Assurance
      (NCQA) are available from NCQA, 2000 L Street NW, Suite 500, Washing-
      ton, DC 20036.

194   For more on quality assurance, see FACCT—The Foundation for Account-
      ability, "Reporting Quality Information to Consumers," a report to the
      Health Care Financing Administration, December 1997, Portland, Oregon.
      Also, C. Bethell and D. Read, "Application of the FACCT Consumer Infor-
      mation Framework to NCQA Data," a report to the National Committee
      for Quality Assurance," March 1998, FACCT—The Foundation for
      Accountability. Or write to: FACCT, 520 SW Sixth Avenue, Suite 700,
      Portland, OR 97204.

195   For more on health insurance matters, see Kimberley Calder and Irene C.
      Card, "Straight Talk about Insurance and Health Plans," in *A Cancer Sur-
      vivor's Almanac*, ed. Barbara Hoffman (Minneapolis: Chronimed, 1996).

12   *The Big Picture*

196   Leo Tolstoy, *The Death of Ivan Ilych* (Chicago: Great Books Foundation,
      1955).

198   Dale Matthews et al., "Religious Commitment and Health Status: A
      Review of the Research and Implications for Family Medicine," *Archives
      of Family Medicine* 7 (March/April 1998): 118–23.
         For more on prayer and healing, see Larry Dossey, *Healing Words: The
      Power of Prayer and the Practice of Medicine* (New York: HarperCollins,
      1993).

199   Rose Elizabeth Bird, Chief Justice of California, Remarks at the First
        Annual Community Forum on Breast Cancer, Los Angeles, May 3, 1980.
          Margaret Craven, *I Heard the Owl Call My Name* (New York: Double-
        day, 1973).
200   Marvella Bayh with Mary Lynn Kotz, *Marvella: A Personal Journey* (New
        York: Harcourt Brace Jovanovich, 1979).
201   Martin Buber, *Good and Evil* (New York: Charles Scribner's Sons, 1952).
202   Hadassah Davis, "My Father, Louis Finkelstein," *Conservative Judaism* 47
        (Summer 1955): 79–90.
209   Terrence Des Pres, *The Survivors: An Anatomy of Life in the Death Camps*
        (Oxford: Oxford University Press, 1976). This is an outstanding account of,
        as the author puts it, "a world ruled by death, but also a world of actual liv-
        ing conditions, of ways of life which are the basis and achievement of life
        in extremity."
          Viktor E. Frankl, *Man's Search for Meaning* (New York: Pocket Books,
        1963).
211   Arthur W. Frank, *The Wounded Storyteller* (Chicago: University of
        Chicago Press, 1995).
213   Primo Levi, *The Reawakening* (New York: Touchstone, 1995).
215   David Saltzman, *The Jester Has Lost His Jingle* (Palos Verdes Estates,
        Calif.: Jester, 1995).

❧ Index

Spingarn, Natalie Davis.
   The new cancer survivors : living with grace, fighting with spirit /
Natalie Davis Spingarn.
       p.   cm.
   Includes bibliographical references and index.
   ISBN 0-8018-6266-3 (alk. paper). — ISBN 0-8018-6267-1 (pbk. :
alk. paper)
       1. Cancer—Popular works.   2. Cancer—Patients.   I. Title.
RC263.S654   1999
362.1´96994—DC21   99-25087
                                                            CIP